ENDING EVIL

ENDING EVIL

How to Heal and Prevent Psychic Illness

Gregory Sweitzer, Psy.D.

Ending Evil: How to Heal and Prevent Psychic Illness
Published by RuthAlan Press

Copyright © 2024 Gregory Alan Sweitzer
All rights reserved.

No portion of this book may be reproduced or transmitted in any form without written permission from the copyright owner, except as permitted by U.S. copyright law.

This book is for information purposes only. A professional relationship has not been established with the reader of this book, and there is no intent to provide professional services to the reader.

ISBN 978-1-7380876-3-1

Contents

Figures and Tables	v
Preface	vii
CHAPTER 1 - The Premise	1
CHAPTER 2 - The Proofs	17
Proof #1: Evidence of Behavior-Borne Virus	18
Proof #2: Evidence of Infection	24
Parasitic manipulation and the benefits of being eaten	27
Proof #3: Evidence of Metabolism	35
Proof #4: Evidence of Growth and Development	40
Proof #5: Evidence of Adaptation	42
Proof #6: Evidence of Reproduction	46
Proof #7: Evidence of Pandemic Spread: Going Viral	57
Proof #8: Evidence of Defenses	62
Proof #9: Evidence of Offensive Strategies and Tactics	69
Back doors to the brain	73
Proof #10: Evidence of Weaponization	79
Baseless conspiracy theories	82
The real conspiracy	83

CHAPTER 3 - Healing — 85

- Become aware of the past in the present — 85
- Believe that change is possible — 86
- Choose to change — 86
- Disengage from psychic illness — 87
- Refocus attention — 88
- Acknowledge participation — 88
- Avoid Judgment — 88
- Let go of the past and get on with your future — 89
- Break the chain — 90
- Change your actions — 90
- Move on — 90
- Deal with real problems, not substitutes — 91
- Make emotions work for you — 92
- Exercise — 92
- Cultivate awareness and understanding — 93
- Respond to your preferences and meet your needs — 94
- Build self-esteem — 94
- Imagine — 94
- Live in the present — 95
- Be open to change — 95
- Pursue goals — 96
- Be flexible — 96
- Think strategically — 98
- Practice skills for dealing with difficult people — 98
- Be honest with yourself — 98
- Recognize your limitations — 99
- Strive — 99
- Laugh — 100
- Create — 100
- Give — 101
- Aspire — 102

Persist ... 102
Assess trustworthiness and take appropriate risks ... 103
Find corrective experiences ... 104
Build healthy relationships ... 104
Simplify ... 105
Choose life ... 107
Love ... 108
Make your world larger ... 109
Practice stewardship ... 111
Cultivate wonder and awe ... 111
Be kind ... 112
Give better than you got ... 113
Follow your dreams ... 113
Choose well ... 113

CHAPTER 4 - Prevention ... 121

Promote responsibility and accountability ... 125
Foster life-promoting values ... 127
The laws of life: using nature to determine healthy values ... 128
Increase public awareness of psychic illness ... 142
Promote equality, opportunity, and justice ... 143
Sell the good life ... 145
Strengthen existing defenses against psychic illness ... 150
Root out corruption ... 156
Increase personal strength and resistance ... 164
   Teach critical thinking and problem-solving ... 164
   Improve coping strategies ... 166
   Teach practical skills for responding to psychic illness ... 170
Outline - How to decrease and prevent psychic illness ... 172
Exploit BBV vulnerabilities ... 177
Disrupt the psychic illness cycle ... 177
Integrate management of behavior-borne viruses ... 179
Make a science of behavioral virology ... 179

Vote with your money	181
Want less, live more	182
Invest in people	183
Reform the economy	189
Restore and protect our natural environment	202

CHAPTER 5 - Crossroads — 207
Love wins — 209

References — 213
About the Author — 221

Figures and Tables

Life Functions of Behavior-Borne Virus	7
Manifestations of Psychic Illness	10-12
Disease Profile	15
The Psychic Illness Cycle	47
STEP 1: Present a Problem	50
STEP 2: Block Resolution of Problem	51
STEP 3: Encourage Pathological Problem-Solving	52
STEP 4: Corrupt	53
Hosts and Vectors of Psychic Illness	56
Healing Psychic Illness	87
Fixed vs. Growth Mindset	97
How to Heal Psychic Illness	117
Psychic Illness is Vulnerable	122

Preface

This book is a summary and extension of *Psychic Illness: The Rise and Fall of Evil on Earth* (Sweitzer, 1988, 1989, 2001). The first edition of *Psychic Illness* was published in 2001. The manuscript for the revised second edition is in preparation. *Psychic Illness* contains additional support for the existence of behavior-borne viruses, background about the prehistoric emergence of psychic illness, a four-chapter catalog of its 171 strategies and tactics, and more comprehensive information about methods for healing and prevention. I recommend you first read *Ending Evil,* and then read the second edition of *Psychic Illness*.

False words are not only evil in themselves, but they infect the soul with evil.
    —Socrates, in Plato's *Phaedo,* circa 360 BC

The evil that afflicts us is not external, it is within us, situated in our very vitals; for that reason, we attain soundness with all the more difficulty, because we do not know that we are diseased.
    —Seneca, *Letters from a Stoic*, L, circa 65 AD

Evil is a disease.
    —William James, *The Varieties of Religious Experience*, Lectures VI and VII: *The Sick Soul*, 1902

Chapter 1

THE PREMISE

I have practiced psychotherapy since 1982, and the problem I see most often is my patients struggling with other people's misbehavior. For over 40 years, I've had a front-row seat to witness the effects of exploitation and abuse. It doesn't take long to figure out that you are often just the clean-up crew, repairing other people's damage after the fact. You learn a lot from putting broken people back together. You learn about what broke them, and how.

Therapists are human naturalists, constantly observing, comparing, cataloging, and hypothesizing. In this environment, steeped in psychopathology, you learn some things. You see some patterns. After a while, the stories start fitting together. The people I see were not born sick. Many of them grew up in sick environments that made them sick, and if they don't get better, they could make other people sick. There is nothing in traditional theories to explain this: psychopathology reproducing through social behavior.

For more than 2,000 years, as far back as Plato and Socrates, people have likened evil to an infectious disease, but none thought the analogy to be anything more than a metaphor. We talk about contagious and corrupting ideologies that spread like a disease. We speak of problems that metastasize and ideas and practices that go viral. We discuss infectious behavior, sick subcultures, crime epidemics, parasitic practices, contaminating influences, toxic people, and we describe the growth of unwanted ideas and behavior as a malignity. And yet, we continue to think of these expressions as only metaphors.

For 36 years (Sweitzer, 1988, 1989, 2001, manuscript in preparation), I have investigated the possibility that evil is a bona fide disease, an infectious problem-solving strategy that can be scientifically described, treated, and prevented. The hypothesis is simple: "Evil is an infectious disease caused by a behavior-borne virus." The hypothesis stands. The proofs are robust, and evidence of the pandemic spread of pathological thinking and behavior is now widespread. This approach to understanding and addressing our oldest and worst problems is more relevant and timely now than when I began this investigation 36 years ago. This disease is spreading. Its problems are intensifying. It has infiltrated our culture, our institutions, our media, and our minds. We are being manipulated and devoured. This is the issue of our age, and if we don't come to terms with it, it will destroy us.

For all our advances in the behavioral sciences, we know appallingly little about why people mistreat each other or how to stop, heal, and prevent it. Considering the magnitude of the problem and the consequences for virtually every area of human life, this ignorance is unacceptable. It seems that we have always struggled to define evil. We have alternately described it as a demonic being, a supernatural force, a philosophical argument, a moral failing, a psychological aberration, a criminal type. And yet, none of these seem quite on the mark. There is another explanation. Perhaps evil is a natural phenomenon, something that evolves over time and preys upon us. Perhaps it is a parasite.

This book presents an admittedly radical and far-reaching hypothesis. This theory provides compelling, scientifically grounded, and empirically testable explanations for many of our worst problems and the extraordinary developments of the past several years, and it yields effective new strategies to address them. The implications for psychology, medicine, religion, history, criminology, public policy, politics, commerce, government, national security, environmental practices, and international relations are profound. What we have long assumed to be inevitable is optional. We are more powerful than we know.

It is not news that people can learn to act in unhealthy ways. What may be surprising is that they are often taught. Far from being "bad habits" that one "picks up" through simple association (Bandura, 1977), many unhealthy activities are the predictable result of systematic social influences orchestrated and carried out against vulnerable people over time. Our problems can take on a life of their own.

It is well established that cultures use cultural transmission to reproduce. Cultures use behavior to pass on a way of life and tell us what we need to know and do to get along in the world. Culture is mental software that runs on biological hardware. We learn from each other, and we teach each other, swimming in a sea of information and instruction. Obviously, some of our behaviors, thoughts, emotions, and beliefs are not helpful. Some are even harmful, but they may be passed on, nonetheless. History is filled with bad ideas and bad practices that caught on and spread. Not infrequently, people pushing these things stand to gain from them, often at other people's expense. Bad ideas and unhealthy practices can be widely adopted, benefitting some while harming others.

When biological organisms are invaded and corrupted, we call it infection. When a mind is invaded and corrupted, it is psychic illness, a communicable disease transmitted through social behavior, including speech. Another word for this is evil. Everything we create can be come infected and turned against us. Psychic illness is caused by a behavior-borne virus (BBV). BBV is not free-living. It resides within its host's mind, using it for its metabolism, activity, growth, and reproduction, making it more like a virus than a bacterium. BBV alters human behavior, thought, emotion, and belief—the four functions of the human psyche. Psychic illness is a behaviorally transmitted disease that lives inside the human mind, commanding us to control others or be controlled. It is a living entity with information and instruction all its own that opposes the purposes of its host. Like many microorganisms, BBV dwells within us, but it is not human. It is alien. We are not possessed, but we are inhabited.

Perhaps the most remarkable thing about evil is that it reproduces. Evil began when someone got stuck on a problem and took it out on others, creating similar issues for them. Since that time, it has tumbled down through the generations, changing as we change, evolving as we evolve. Psychic illness is predictable. It follows patterns. It has an observable life cycle and a describable process of transmission. It is passed between individuals in a four-part life cycle: engage, confuse, weaken, corrupt. It harms us mentally emotionally, and spiritually, and makes our behavior poisonous. Evil need not be mysterious. It is a common, tangible, knowable condition transmitted through social behavior. Once we understand this, we see it is also vulnerable to the tools of science and may be eradicated.

Evil is not a supernatural force. Evil is a natural phenomenon that can be defined, described, and addressed by science (Watson, 1995). It has been fashioned into weaponized tools that are increasingly used against us by nefarious actors with devastating effects. Older than history but younger than humans, it has obscured its presence and eluded detection. A cunning and stealthy adversary, it has operated for ages without our understanding what it is or how it works. This ends now.

In biology, infectious agents must have some material, tangible cell or substance that causes the infection. So where is it? Psychic illness is a cultural creation. It has no independent physical structure. It is a mind virus transmitted by social behavior. It is psychogenic, a disorder of function, not structure, a malfunctioning of the mass of our brain cells, acting in concert, which individually may be normal and healthy. Psychic illness uses cultural transmission for infection. It uses behavior. Behavior is one of its vulnerabilities, for behavior exposes internal mental processes, and behavior transmits behavior-borne virus. In my work, I have described 171 behavioral strategies, tactics, and defenses employed by psychic illness and detailed its life cycle (Sweitzer, 1988, 1989, 2001, and manuscript in preparation).

Behavior-borne virus is housed within the brain, which serves as a biological substrate. BBV seizes control and makes our minds work against us. In much the same way, computers can house a collection of magnetic charges on a disk—a substrate—and those charges can constitute an effective computer virus. The common cold infects through person-to-person contact; computer viruses infect through computer-to-computer contact: infected attachments, downloaded apps, and flash drives. Viruses can and do exist outside of biology. There is precedent for this.

Infectious disease is organized information and instruction that invades and alters the functioning of another organism. It is one organism imposing its plan upon another. Physical structure is not required for infection. Tangible microbes with physical structure are a common but not exclusive means to this end. They are a vehicle, one type of vehicle. There are others. It is time to expand the concept of infectious disease to include pathological information and instruction communicated through behavior.

While the concept of a behavior-borne virus is unorthodox, our understanding of infectious disease has changed over time, and it continues to evolve. Ancient Greece, Rome, India, and Judea had primitive notions of infection, such as the miasma theory put forth by Hippocrates (400 B.C.E.), but they lacked the technical means

> **LIFE FUNCTIONS OF
> BEHAVIOR-BORNE VIRUS**
>
> **Metabolism**: BBV feeds on energy diverted from thwarted needs and drives, energy released from the damaging and breaking of human relationships, and resources extracted from its prey.
>
> **Activity**: Upon exposure to a candidate psyche, BBV initiates engagement, confusion, weakening, and corruption tactics. These are described in detail in eponymous chapters Three through Six of *Psychic Illness*.
>
> **Growth**: BBV plants itself in the unconscious mind, takes root, and progressively controls behavior, thought, emotion, and belief to complete successive stages of the psychic illness cycle. If not stopped, it eventually brings the infected individual to the mature corruption phase of the illness (transmit or self-destruct).
>
> **Reproduction**: BBV engages, infects, and reproduces through social behavior.

to identify the agents of infection. During the 17th and 18th centuries, improvements in optics and the invention of the microscope led to the direct observation of microorganisms and the gradual adoption of the germ theory of disease. Viruses were added to germ theory in 1892 when Dmitry Ivanovsky discovered that agents far smaller than bacteria could cause infectious diseases. When specific microorganisms were first linked to individual diseases, pathologists were excited by their newfound ability to identify pathogens responsible for longstanding afflictions such as anthrax, plague, malaria, tuberculosis, and cholera. This spurred the new science of epidemiology. Prevention was initially thought to be simply a matter of avoiding exposure to pathogenic organisms. Now we know better.

After learning that we are regularly exposed to virulent pathogens without developing symptoms, we expanded germ theory to include other considerations in the development of illness, and we've since identified numerous intervening variables that affect the disease process. Genetic, immunological, developmental, nutritional, environmental, and situational factors—including exposure to stressful life situations and one's mental and emotional state—influence the course of illnesses such as cancer, cardiovascular disease, diabetes mellitus, gastrointestinal disorders, immunological disorders, multiple sclerosis, psoriasis, arthritis, and bacteriological and viral infection. The functioning and health of all human organs and systems are affected by experiential factors, and even the physical, structural development of the human brain is altered by life experience (Perry, 2001).

When first put forth, germ theory described a simple cause-and-effect relationship between microbes and infectious diseases. Now we examine health within the context of an individual's social environment, their thought process, and emotional functioning. It does not require a great leap of the imagination to progress from accepting that experiential factors can influence illness to recognizing that they can contain, carry, and cause illness. Furthermore, we know that people can become addicted and lose control to culturally engineered activities such as gambling, collecting, shopping, gaming, and viewing pornography and social media, demonstrating that artificial, specifically crafted cultural experiences can systematically and reliably seize control of the psyche, extract resources, and harm one's health. Information and instruction are the only requirements for invasion and control, and they may be housed in mediums other than biology.

The mind exists solely inside biological organs: our brain, nervous system, and body. It has no other material existence. And yet, the mind directs behavior, it communicates with other minds, and it builds civilizations. The mind is quite real. The mind can change itself and its environment in profound ways. Minds are also susceptible to mental illness, and minds can change other minds. There is really nothing to prevent minds from housing a type of mental illness that they communicate to other minds through social behavior. Teaching and learning happen all the time. If you want to fundamentally understand something, examine what it does, how it functions. This tells you more about the essence of a thing than the materials it is made of.

For those who cannot accept that evil is a virus, the ideas presented here are equally valid when conceived as a social learning theory describing a form of social contagion. From this perspective, evil is simply a set of unhealthy lessons taught by one person and adopted by others, concepts that are entirely compatible with the theory of behavioral virology. The main tenets are unaffected. Whether we call this a behavior-borne virus (BBV) or social learning is a question of semantics. It must be noted, however, that these "lessons" exhibit some very peculiar characteristics. They seize control, steal energy, and multiply. They use camouflage to evade detection and illicitly transfer resources from the "learner" to the "teacher." Such activities are more often associated with parasites than with social instruction. However, if you feel more comfortable using the terminology of social learning, so be it. The terms are not important; the ideas are.

Evil seeks to exploit or harm the living for illicit gain or unwholesome gratification. It is often a substantial factor in (this is an incomplete list):

abuse
addiction
animal cruelty
anti-Semitism
assault
authoritarianism
bigotry
blackmail
brainwashing
bullying
cheating
child abuse
child pornography
class systems
coercion
colonialism

computer malware
corruption
crime
cult indoctrination
cutting
deception
defamation
denialism
despotism
dictatorship
discrimination
disease burden
dishonesty
divisive rhetoric
domestic violence
elder abuse

elitism
environmental
  degradation
ethnic cleansing
exploitation
extremism
fake news
false imprisonment
false/manipulative
  advertising
fascism
firearm deaths
fraud
gaslighting
genocide
gossip
greed
harassment
hate speech & crimes
homelessness
human trafficking
imperialism
incest
indentured servitude
inequality
injustice
intentional trauma
intolerance

kidnapping
lying
maltreatment
manipulative and
  controlling behavior
media-induced
  trauma
misinformation
murder
nationalism
neglect
oppression
organized crime
police brutality
pollution
poverty
prejudice
propaganda
psychological warfare
racism
radicalization
revenge
revisionism
rumor
sadomasochism
self-defeating
  behavior
sexism

sexual assault
slander
slavery
stalking
substance abuse
suicide
systemic privilege
terrorism
torture
totalitarianism
toxic relationships
trauma (intentional)
tribalism
vandalism
violence
war

These problems are one problem, symptoms of a single disease wearing many masks. Notice they all involve behavior. Behavior is how psychic illness is transmitted. This is abuse on a social scale.

Synonymous with the mind, the psyche consists of the functions of the brain and nervous system, including thought, emotion, and belief, interacting with their environment through behavior. A unit of culture, the psyche is determined by heredity, experience, and choice.

Psychic illness is learned and taught through purposeful and systematic behavior in unhealthy relationships, internalized as a personal set of strategies for achieving goals and solving problems, and repeated in future interactions with others. Psychic illness is transmitted by frustrating drives and creating artificial conflicts between the receiver's needs, confusing and weakening the receiver, defeating defenses the receiver might employ to cope with the situation, and encouraging their replacement with pathological activity.

~ ~ ~

Reading the news, it would seem that the world is filled with senseless harm and destruction, enormously degrading our quality of life. Is this inevitable, or are we living below our potential? Is it human nature for people to take advantage, exploit, abuse, and wreck each other? Is this normal? Is this who we are? Or are there identifiable influences that foster and encourage such behavior, influences that can be modified, reduced, and eliminated? Is it possible to develop a science of good and evil?

For too long, we have imagined evil to be a mysterious bogeyman, something unknowable and unassailable. This has allowed it to operate largely unaddressed and unchecked. By defining evil as a supernatural force, we have shrouded it in mystery and prevented serious discussion and effective action. Evil is real. Its actions are observable. Its effects are tangible. Evil manifests as a describable and predictable condition transmitted through social behavior. When we recognize evil as a disease, we can use science to combat it. Suddenly, we can diagnose, research, prevent, and treat many of our oldest and worst problems. The disease model allows us to reveal its operations, disrupt its life cycle, and heal using established, off-the-shelf epidemiological methods, public health strategies, and psychological treatments. Evil is more vulnerable, and we are more powerful, than we ever dreamed.

Behavior-borne viruses are real. Hijacking the enormous power of culture, they can be far more dangerous than biological viruses. These foreign agents turn human thinking, emotions, beliefs, and behavior against us. They can cause people to believe outrageous lies, regardless of reason and fact, and act irrationally and destructively, even against their own interests. When BBV is allowed to run its course and operate unopposed, it causes mental, emotional, moral, and behavioral deterioration. It brings about social conflict, resource squandering, environmental and economic deterioration, civil unrest, violence, war, and systemic (economic, political, social, ecosystem, population, and civilization) collapse. This virus is rapacious. Aliens have invaded, and we have responded not by uniting but by tearing each other apart. This changes when we see these things for what they are. Other people are not the enemy. The virus is. Wake up.

We live in a time of great peril and equally great opportunity. What sort of world do we wish to inhabit? We have everything we need. Our cultures and institutions must change their values and actions to better align with the laws of life. These are opportunities to effect dramatic changes at critical moments in disrupted lives. Treating psychic illness is not complicated. Preventing it is not expensive. Evil costs. Given the enormous lost opportunities and wasted resources, addressing psychic illness yields an enormous bonanza. It is expensive *not* to address it. This is not a question of resources or technology; it is a question of resolve.

Serious problems confront us, but we can do amazing things when we work together. We can study the ways of this strange illness, map and chart its workings, and plan a better way. We can expose evil as a fraud and begin dismantling it. We can stop rewarding psychic illness in our institutions, make better use of healthy incentives, decrease its access to media and vulnerable persons, and teach people effective skills and strategies for recognizing and responding to it. Our task now is to choose between the very different paths available to us.

DISEASE PROFILE	
Name:	Psychic Illness
Pathogen:	Behavior-borne virus (BBV)
Host species:	Human beings
Points of entry:	Senses of sight, sound, touch, taste, and smell.
Hosts/Vectors:	The human mind, culture, subcultures, institutions, families, media, and electronic devices.
Mode of transmission:	Behavior, including speech.
Susceptible hosts:	Isolated, dependent, and weakened individuals with depleted resources, deficient resistance, immature defenses, undeveloped morality, and lacking acquired immunity.
Reproduction:	Behavioral transmission and exploitation of the host's resources to compel reproduction. The four-part life cycle includes engage, confuse, weaken, and corrupt.
Pathogenesis:	Diversion and depletion of resources, resulting in problematic thoughts, emotions, behavior, and beliefs.
Immune response:	Formation of norms, mores, rules-based behavior, spiritual beliefs, and a variety of egalitarian institutions, cooperative endeavors, banding together, and other practices evolved to protect against predation.

> If you do not seek scientific proof that evil is a behavior-borne virus, advance to Chapter Three, *Healing*.

Chapter 2

THE PROOFS

> An extraordinary claim requires extraordinary proof.
> —Marcello Truzzi

The proof that evil is an infectious disease caused by a behavior-borne virus is in 10 parts.

1. Evidence of behavior-borne virus
2. Evidence of infection
3. Evidence of metabolism
4. Evidence of growth and development
5. Evidence of adaptation
6. Evidence of reproduction
7. Evidence of pandemic spread
8. Evidence of defenses
9. Evidence of offensive strategies and tactics
10. Evidence of weaponization

Proof #1: Evidence of Behavior-Borne Virus

Must infectious agents be confined to cells, nucleic acids, and proteins? Or can viruses also exist as information and instruction housed in minds and transmitted through behavior? A computer virus can exist as an idea in a programmer's brain, spoken words, finger taps on a keyboard, electrons streaming through a copper wire, photons beamed through fiber optic cable, magnetized sections of a storage disk, tape, or integrated circuit, or as ink printed on paper. Things transmitted by behavior are shapeshifters because we have developed numerous technologies to store and communicate thoughts and data. This doesn't make behavior-borne viruses incorporeal; it just makes them different from what we're used to. They live in minds, media, institutions, cultures, and computers, not cells.

The essence of infection is invasion and exploitation by an external force. It is one organism replacing another's plans with its own. Consider the biological virus. Little more than encoded information and instruction, the biological virus is the stripped-down, bare-bones version of life, approaching the absolute minimum for biological replication. It has found advantage in manipulating and exploiting other organisms' genetic transmission for its own ends, commandeering a host's mitotic cellular reproduction. It physically invades and overrules its host's genetic code, substituting its plan. Biological viruses are curious things, unlike other life forms. They look like crystals under a microscope and contain only particles of DNA or RNA enclosed in a protein coat. The sole purpose of their physical structure is to house data and provide a means of implanting it in other organisms. Biological viruses are not free-living. On their own, they lay dormant, exhibiting no metabolism, activity, growth, or reproduction—four functions of life. They cannot reproduce outside a living cell of another organism. Once activated by the presence of a host, they must invade and use the host's cellular machinery for their metabolism and reproduction. Biological viruses teach us that the size of an organism does not correspond to its ability to cause disease. Mass does not correlate with illness; information and instruction do.

Biologists have found even smaller infectious agents called subviruses, the simplest infectious agents known. Perhaps the most interesting subviruses are prions, tiny infectious particles consisting only of a single protein. Prions contain no nucleic acid, DNA, or RNA. Prions have been implicated in scrapie in sheep, and in humans, they cause bovine spongiform encephalopathy (BSE or mad cow disease), kuru, fatal familial insomnia (FFI), and Creutzfeldt-Jakob Disease (CJD). A prion's information and instruction are limited to the organizational structure of its protein, an example of biological infectious self-replication occurring even without nucleic acid. Prions may not be alive in a traditional sense, but they do infect, reproduce, neutralize defenses, and cause disease and death. The discoveries of microscopic multicellular and unicellular organisms, bacteria, viruses, and subviruses have expanded our concept of infectious disease and blurred the boundaries between animate and inanimate matter.

Viruses are parasites, and parasites have always been our worst enemies, having killed far more of us than predatory animals and other humans combined. Microbial parasites are all the more dangerous due to their small size, large numbers, and phenomenally fast reproduction and adaptation. Viruses strip it down even more, containing only bits of RNA or DNA sheathed in protein. Behavior-borne virus goes one better, outsourcing even its physical structure. It has no bones, body, or even genes; it depends entirely upon its host for tangible infrastructure. This is economy and stealth on steroids, the ultimate virus.

Biological viruses are wildly successful, found in every species on the planet, even in bacteria and fungi. They are Earth's most persistent and prevalent life forms. They are found everywhere, in incredible numbers. A typical liter of seawater contains more than 10 billion virus particles. All living things carry viruses in their cells, and for every human cell in your body, you house 100 virus particles (Mokili, Rohwer, et al., 2012). Nearly half of our DNA came from viruses that infected our ancestors' sperm and egg cells. And yet, most microbiologists do not classify biological viruses as true living organisms, citing their dependence upon their hosts for metabolism and reproduction. For the purposes of our argument, however, this is a moot point. Even if viruses are not considered to be alive, that does not negate our hypothesis that evil is a (viral) disease. Alive or not alive, it is well established that viruses exhibit Darwinian evolution, and they can and often do cause disease. Call them what you will; they are coming for us.

There are more parasitic species than nonparasitic species. Parasitism is the rule, not the exception; it is Earth's most common and successful survival strategy. There is nothing to exempt cultural transmission from carrying parasitic viral disease. Nature abhors an unexploited niche. It may be inevitable that all forms of transmission—biological, electronic, and cultural—eventually become vulnerable to corrupted information and instruction capable of reproduction. We've just created computers, and already they are stricken by electronic viruses. Computer systems can be infected and corrupted by digital parasites that hijack their host's software and hardware and turn it to their purposes. Stephen Hawking described computer viruses as living parasites that exploit the metabolism of the computers they infect and replicate in their memory (Hawking, 1996). Some computer viruses can even mutate. If computers can host mutating viruses and become diseased and infectious, then why not cultures and psyches?

Viruses have four basic tasks:
1. Seize control.
2. Supplant the host's information and instruction.
3. Exploit the host's resources for their own benefit.
4. Compel reproduction.

Interpersonal behavior is quite capable of accomplishing the first three tasks. In humans, this is common. This leaves us with one issue: Can behaviorally transmitted information and instruction compel its own reproduction?

In 1893, Sigmund Freud described repetition compulsion as the urge, driven by unresolved unconscious conflicts, to repeat traumatic events from one's past (van der Kolk, 1989). In 1976, Richard Dawkins introduced the idea of memes, units of cultural information that routinely pass from one mind to another. Humans are wired for mimicry; we have inborn instincts to imitate and learn. Doing what others do comes naturally to us. Compelling reproduction is easy. Monkey see, monkey do. People also choose psychic illness out of pain and desperation. They choose it because they lack alternatives for relief. Reproduction is compelled because it relieves pain. Corrupt choices can also be gratifying; the person may choose them because they feel good. Reproduction is compelled because it brings pleasure.

~ ~ ~

Let's talk about choice. Recall that biological evolution uses natural selection to guide life. Genes mutate randomly, and organisms possessing beneficial changes are slightly more likely to last. Natural selection needs many generations to adapt, making it very slow. Life's difficulty adapting to rapidly changing circumstances caused Earth's mass extinctions: each was preceded by sudden, vast, untypical environmental changes.

During the Ice Age, for nearly three million years, the environments we inhabited were unstable, in near-constant flux. They changed rapidly and repeatedly, stressing all organisms. We invented culture to cope with that flux. Culture allows us to change very quickly. To accomplish this, culture uses artificial selection (choice) for guidance, making it much faster than natural selection. Using culture, we can make intelligent trials, immediately evaluate the results, choose and adopt improved practices, and teach better ways of doing things to others. Culture adapts much faster than natural selection by using choice.

But there's the rub. Artificial selection requires that we participate in and guide the course of our evolution. Culture and choice gave us incredible new powers, but they also introduced new vulnerabilities. We could now make poor choices, unhealthy, harmful, and corrupt choices, and we could teach these to others. We could carry new forms of disease—corrupted information and instruction. Of course, we could also make good and healthy choices that benefit all and elevate us. We could choose good as well as evil. Faced with these choices, we discovered values and spirituality. Using behavior to transmit life's information and instruction created new opportunities for disease. It exposed the mind to the possibility of organized and systematic unhealthy influences, things we had to wrestle with and adapt to. It also brought the possibility of our becoming something better than we had been. We developed a sense of right and wrong and became moral.

Choosing, learning, and teaching also favor intelligence, so we gradually evolved to become more intelligent. Cultural transmission made us moral and smart. Choice has always been our greatest power and our greatest vulnerability. Our choices changed us into something fundamentally different from what we had been. We participated in our evolution and became human beings. Life had never done this before. We continue to choose and change, and there is no telling what we will become.

Psychic illness, evil, is a behavior-borne virus, the natural result of life reaching out and flowing into all available cracks and corners, wherever it finds suitable places to inhabit and resources to exploit. It is a parasitic viral disease, every bit as much as rabies, smallpox, and polio. There is, however, one overriding difference. Psychic illness requires our consent and cooperation. It requires our participation. It requires our choice.

Proof #2: Evidence of Infection

We are born innocent, but we don't die innocent. Something happens to us between birth and death. Something changes us. Evil works on a person. It manufactures problems and creates artificial conflicts to confuse and weaken us. It frustrates our needs, blocks our drives, defeats our defenses, and thwarts our efforts to solve its dilemmas. Or it spoils and indulges us, so we don't develop properly and become weak and corrupted, learning to meet our needs at other people's expense. Psychic illness diverts energies meant to address problems and turns them against us. It obstructs, entices, and encourages people to choose sick substitutes. This is a squeeze play. How we cope with these problems becomes a set style for interacting with our environment, continuing long after these first problems have passed.

The provocative and engaging activities of psychic illness, followed by altered behavior, thinking, emotions, and beliefs, are evidence of infection. Infection begins with engagement, the establishment and maintenance of an unhealthy relationship. Pain, problems, and vice are the primary engagement tools of psychic illness, the catalysts that engage us and stimulate action for pathological relief or pleasure. Pain and pleasure draw our attention to problems and opportunities, and they motivate us to act. Threats of pain and promises of pleasure trigger biological changes that push us to vigorous action. Bypassing the brain's cortex and activating the limbic system, pain and pleasure can commandeer our behavior, thoughts, emotions, and beliefs regardless of our conscious interpretations and decisions (Rainville et al., 1997).

The transmitter frustrates, seduces, baits, injures, and provokes; he encourages vice and addiction, doing whatever he can to involve others in his psychopathology. Even isolated acts can incite powerful emotions of fear, anger, hate, and desire that initiate and maintain engagement. Threats, physical harm, loss, pain, and disfigurement also involve us. Alternatively, spoiling a receiver makes him desirous and lazy, prone to vice for gratification and becoming dishonest, manipulative, and controlling with others to satisfy his desires. Prevented from resolving problems in healthy ways, if he makes unhealthy choices, the receiver can become infected just struggling to free himself.

The uneven distribution of psychic illness within populations is evidence of infection. Psychic illness is clustered by person, place, and time. It occurs more frequently and is concentrated around particular individuals and groups. Some people encounter little of it, while for others, it is a frequent companion. Bad actors leave a trail of wrecked and broken people in their wake, and some families, worksites, and political systems are rife with it. This clustering of psychic illness by time and place provides evidence that it is fed and restrained by environmental factors, including exposure. It is also well-established that many traumas, such as domestic violence, addiction, child abuse, and neglect, are frequently intergenerational. They can be taught and learned—transmitted. Exposure creates risk, and this is evidence of infection. The persistence of psychic illness, often for entire lifetimes, also suggests that it changes people in ways that make it difficult for them to change back. Such profoundly dysfunctional and lasting change in response to exposure is not natural. It is evidence of infection.

Psychic illness infests us with parasitic ideas and practices. It encourages and incentivizes all manner of vice and illicit pleasures. Vice alters and degrades people, preparing them to exploit and harm. Vice is the advance army of psychic illness, engaging and softening a population, changing the rules, and making evil acceptable. Greed is not good; greed is gross. Vice transfers control to the virus and extracts human resources to feed.

Psychic illness is taught and learned within relationships. Relationships are the arena where unhealthy behaviors, thoughts, emotions, and choices are taught, practiced, and perfected. Psychic illness may be learned within any relationship, but it is most active in sustained relationships with significant psychic exchange: between parent and child, partners, siblings, co-workers, and friends. It is also found in relationships between acquaintances and even strangers. Although psychic illness may be expressed in single encounters, it is more effectively transmitted in enduring relationships. Brutal, single-event experiences, such as rape, robbery, assault, and kidnapping, do traumatize and engage a receiver, but they seldom result in learning that compels him to repeat the experience. In longer-term relationships, the pathology tends to be more subtle and hidden. Whatever the relationship, the receiver must become involved with the transmitter. He must be engaged.

Psychically ill relationships are often characterized by unequal power between the transmitter and receiver and a struggle for control. A troublemaker by trade, the transmitter creates problems to engage the receiver. He is planting problems to harvest pain. These are not normal problems; they are artificial, manufactured frustrations tailored to the situation. These dilemmas are difficult to avoid, easy to engage, hard to leave, and nearly impossible to solve. This is a sore that cannot heal. The controlling transmitter is sick and needs to change, but instead of changing, he works on the receiver, exploits her vulnerabilities, and thwarts her growth. He gets *her* to change.

Parasitic Manipulation and the Benefits of Being Eaten

Parasites often alter host behavior to increase their chances of survival, and behavior-altering parasites are surprisingly common. Few things are more frightening than the thought of an alien organism taking over your brain and making you *do things*, but many parasites do just that, manipulating their host's nervous system and altering their behavior and cognition, effectively turning their hosts into zombies to further their own reproduction. These include various flukes (Zimmer, 2000), hairworms, guinea worms (which infect humans), ichneumon wasps, emerald cockroach wasps, jewel wasps, the fungus Ophiocordyceps unilateralis, and many others. Once infected, the host's behavior may become pathological and self-defeating, even suicidal, to serve the purposes of the parasite. These puppeteer parasites can wipe out entire host populations, subsiding only when there is nothing left for them to feed on.

The emerging science of neuroparasitology investigates these parasites and how they change their host's nervous system, behavior, and cognition (Libersat, Kaiser, et al., 2018). In extreme forms, these brain-manipulating parasites can cause suicidal behavior in affected hosts who eagerly offer themselves to predators for ingestion. Infected hosts alert predators by leaving cover, acting conspicuous, careless, or erratic, darting about, and rushing into situations that make them available and visible, inviting their demise. This kills the host but benefits the parasite by allowing it to infect another animal.

Nature provides many examples of parasitic manipulation. Infected fish swim to the water's surface and turn their white bellies to the sky, attracting predatory birds. Infected black pill bugs migrate to white surfaces, making them more visible to predators. Infected crickets are attracted to light, bringing them to open, watery areas where they are eaten by fish. Infected ants climb to the tips of blades of grass, where they wait to be eaten by grazing animals. Moniliformis moniliformis causes the common cockroach to dart about a room when suddenly exposed to light, making it more likely to be noticed and eaten by a rat—all the better for the parasite, which needs to spend its adult life inside rat intestines. When lyssavirus, the virus that causes rabies, enters an infected dog's brain, it increases salivation that is loaded with virus particles and provokes a compulsion to bite, transmitting the virus to a new host. Rabies-caused hydrophobia also decreases a dog's drinking, causing dehydration that concentrates the virus in saliva, making it more infectious. Some hosts are tranquilized, making them incautious and prone to risk-taking. These changes in decision-making and behavior are accomplished by altering hormones and neurotransmitters, injecting neurotoxins, and directly invading brain circuits. The effect is up-regulation and down-regulation of specific behaviors (Ibid.), increasing or decreasing the likelihood that they occur in the presence of certain stimuli.

It is unsurprising that parasites should drug their prey—it is an old trick to gain control and take advantage. What makes these manipulating parasites stand out is their ability to turn hosts into zombies—intermediate hosts that offer themselves up to be eaten by yet another host, inside which the parasite can complete its life cycle. For many parasites, there are benefits to being eaten. This strategy is beyond the typical smash-and-grab of seizing control and stealing resources. It alters the host's behavior, puts it to work for the parasite, and turns it into a collaborator. This is higher-level parasitism, and it means we cannot always assume that animals or people are acting entirely of their own volition. Persons infected with BBV can exhibit this same zombie-like process in the corruption phase of the disease when controlled receivers allow others to exploit or harm them.

Most parasite manipulations are less dramatic, stopping short of compelling suicide or self-harm and instead cause the host to spread infection. In humans, several skin conditions create itchy pustules filled with infectious fluid, the scratching of which releases microorganisms into the environment where they can find new hosts. Intestinal viruses stimulate increased fecal volume, pressure, and activity in the form of watery, spraying diarrhea loaded with infectious particles, more effectively dispersing them into the environment. The plasmodium that causes malaria and the virus that causes dengue fever alter human body odor, making us more attractive to mosquitoes. Respiratory infections, such as the common cold, routinely cause coughing, sniffling, and sneezing—behaviors that discharge virus particles into our environment. Our gut bacteria influence our emotions, diet, and behavior (Trevelline and Kohl, 2022). Infection-changed behavior is so common and predictable that physicians routinely recognize many altered human behaviors as reliable signs of infectious disease. We are moved, perhaps more than we know, by parasites.

Biological parasites can even alter our thinking. *Toxoplasma gondii*, an obligate protozoan parasite known to induce changes in the behavior of its hosts, is found in 20-80% of humans. T. gondii has been associated with decreased superego strength or conscience (Flegr, Zitková, et al., 1996), a decreased willingness to accept group moral standards (Ibid.), increased risk-taking, increased entrepreneurial activity (Johnson, 2018), road rage (Desmettre, 2020), and suicidal thought and attempts (Ibid.). T. gondii infection has also been investigated as a possible risk factor for schizophrenia (Torrey, E. F. et al., 2012).

Behavior-borne virus, the infectious agent that causes psychic illness, is a mind-altering, behavior-changing parasite. It seizes control of the host's cognitive, emotional, moral, and behavioral circuits and compels reproduction through altered social behavior. When people repeatedly do things that are irrational, harmful, and patently against their interests; when you can identify an involved actor that gains from or is gratified by this; and when this same actor suggested, instructed, or encouraged this type of behavior; this is evidence of infection and parasite-changed behavior.

Examples of infection-induced disadvantageous behavior in humans abound. Consider people's refusal of free and effective vaccination during a deadly pandemic. During COVID-19, more than one person insisted they preferred death to vaccination, and for many, that became their fate. To many, the stated reasons for vaccine refusal appeared remarkably weak. Citing health and safety concerns while refusing effective inoculation during a pandemic is unhealthy and unsafe behavior. Citing freedom as one's reason for declining the offer of a voluntary vaccine makes little sense when one can scarcely imagine outcomes more confining than long COVID and death. People have the right to make their own health choices, but if the dissemination of false information about the COVID-19 virus and vaccine was motivated by political and economic gain, and if refusing vaccination harmed and killed people, this is a problem.

Vaccine refusers were told that something important (e.g., their freedom) was being taken from them. This is a known, commonly used tactic to incite fear, disable reason, and stimulate pathological behavior. If the persons who told them this profited from doing so, e.g., through more followers, ratings, advertising dollars, or political power and control, this is also a problem.

Psychic illness is bold. This drama played out in slow motion in broad daylight for power and profit, using infected media and politicians as weapons. Anti-vaccine thinking and behavior during a deadly pandemic are similar to the behavior exhibited by suicide cults. In each instance, people die abetted by sick individuals for personal profit and political gain. And for some, unhealthy gratification. The spread of vaccine denialism during the COVID-19 pandemic enriched and empowered persons who peddled disinformation. These were schemes for making money and obtaining votes. Media can be used as vectors: contaminated, dangerous, and unaccountable. Irresponsible disinformation poisons a society, and our stacking bodies a million high tells us something must be done.

Beware of who you listen to and the stories you tell yourself. There are stories that can put you into a body bag.

Another example of mass behavioral infection causing disadvantageous behavior is found in American politics, which for the past 40 years has increasingly been characterized by a growing number of voters choosing candidates and positions that clearly work against their interests (Frank, 2004). Beginning in the 1980s, conservative politicians and media, lacking popular support, skillfully shifted political discourse away from people's lived quality of life (i.e., the tangible impact of representatives' actions upon their constituents' lives) to divisive and emotionally charged "hot button" ideological wedge issues (e.g., race, religion, abortion, gun rights, and environmental, immigration, and gender issues).

Conservative politicians and media ridiculed those who disagreed with them and engaged in emotional disinformation campaigns filled with false and demeaning personal attacks (e.g., dirty hippies, welfare queens, draft dodgers, tree huggers, and pedophile groomers) that mischaracterized those they attacked. Avoiding facts because they cannot win on the merits of their positions, they instead result to ad hominem attacks. Distract, divide, conquer. It worked. People stopped talking about how their representatives' actions impacted their lived quality of life and focused instead on identity politics and culture wars. Divide and conquer. In the United States, commitment to this radically conservative ideology now often surpasses even people's loyalty to their country, its foundational principles of democracy, and checks and balances on power. These same tactics were used by Adolf Hitler. We have become a shadow of our former selves.

The strategy and objectives of the higher-level instigators of all this were more nuanced and considered than the rank-and-file, but still quite simple: encourage grievance-collecting. Make people afraid, angry, and distracted. Play to their base emotions and then *quietly cart off the prizes of wealth and power when no one is looking.* People fell for it. Conservative American voters signed on to and enthusiastically supported the largest transfer of wealth and power in the history of the United States at a staggering cost to themselves. The Great Siphoning—implementation of supply-side "trickle-down" economics—tipped the scales to enormously enrich the wealthiest and most powerful in society at great cost to those who voted for it.

The results have been devastating. Since the 1970s, inflation-adjusted incomes for most people in America have remained flat even though their economic productivity and output *doubled*. Those productivity gains were siphoned off by the wealthy, dramatically increasing their fortunes. During this time, the costs of food, fuel, housing, education, healthcare, and retirement all soared. Lack of opportunity, poverty, inequality, homelessness, and political instability have become hugely problematic. Bare necessities of housing, water, education, clean air, and physical security can no longer be taken for granted. As more people are pushed out of the middle class, we are becoming a tiered society. And yet, this radical brand of conservatism remains politically viable in America. Clearly, something other than reason, reward, altruism, principle, or self-interest is at work here.

We are being played. For decades, we've been told that "government is the problem," "greed is good," and that lowering taxes on the wealthy would "trickle down" via the supposed magic of supply-side economics (George H.W. Bush, a Republican, famously called it "voodoo economics") to the rest of us. It didn't happen. At the same time, in utter hypocrisy, we were also told that economic and social measures *to benefit most people in our society* "wouldn't work," and such actions were demonized as socialism. Miniscule adjustments to keep the poor from losing their homes and starving were derided as welfare. In other words, the smart and moral thing to do is to take money from people who need it and give it to people who don't. This Orwellian doublespeak translates to "poverty is wealth." Let's take a look at how this nonsense is sold.

Reason is an evolved ability, hundreds of millions of years younger than emotion. When stressed, the brain reverts to its default: automatic emotional responses simplify and speed up decision-making but increase the probability of error. Irrational and emotionally manipulative appeals to primitive and base emotions—such as insecurity, fear, anger, disgust, and outrage—are crafted to bypass our neocortex, reason, and logic. They head straight for our "lizard brain"—ancient emotional circuits that react strongly and violently when we fear something important is being taken from us. Try removing a food-insecure dog's dish when it is eating and watch the dramatic transformation as these circuits are activated. People who are afraid are easy to manipulate and control. We are being treated like dogs, and it is working.

The urge to prey upon, exploit, attack, harm, and kill members of one's own species, one's own pack, one's own family, one's own children, one's own future, one's own financial interests, or oneself, is entirely unnatural, contrary to our interests, and detrimental to our survival and reproduction. This is not normal behavior. This is evidence of infection. There can be no other explanation.

When a person repeatedly acts against their own self-interest, when external actors have communicated instructions to this effect, and when those who encourage this behavior stand to gain from or are gratified by this, think infection. Think virus. There is a good chance the person's thoughts and behavior have been hijacked, and they have fallen under the control of an external actor, an alien influence.

Proof #3: Evidence of Metabolism

Psychic illness has a parasitic metabolism, draining people of resources it uses to operate. In atomic and chemical systems—in atoms and molecules—energy is stored in connections between the parts of the system. This energy maintains bonds that hold the system together and allow it to last. Breaking connections holding those parts together releases energy stored within those bonds. This is true in physics (e.g., nuclear reaction) and chemistry (e.g., chemical reaction). Nuclear power plants use nuclear reactions—they break atomic bonds—to feed electrical grids. Biological organisms use chemical reactions—they break chemical bonds—to feed bodies.

We humans invest and store our energy in social-emotional bonds we call attachments. Attachments contain the energy from emotional investments we make in each other over time. These emotional bonds hold relationships, families, and cultures together. Psychic illness damages and severs these relationships and feeds off the released emotional pain. It divides people and destroys what we care about and are invested in. It breaks bonds by exploiting, alienating, abusing, dividing, harming, and killing people. It is a destructor, a parasitic metabolizer of life and living relationships, a destroyer of all that is good and true and noble in the world. It feeds on emotional pain. Cruelty is not an unintended by-product of psychic illness. Cruelty is the point.

Goodness and evil are scientifically valid constructs with tangible properties and palpable consequences for all that lives (Watson, 1995). Goodness promotes systemic survival; evil causes systemic destruction. Goodness forms reciprocal connections and stores energy in those connections; evil is a parasite that divides people by damaging and breaking bonds and then feeds off the released energy and stolen resources. The study of the formation and severing of living relationships is the study of goodness and evil.

Psychic illness metabolizes not only our relationships; it also taps into and manipulates our needs and drives, turning them against us to stimulate pathological thinking and behavior. When we cannot meet our needs in healthy ways, we may be tempted to meet them in unhealthy ways, to take our problems out on others and turn to vice or other self-defeating, destructive, and acting-out behavior. The transmitter engages and weakens the receiver by frustrating her needs, thwarting her drives, and encouraging life-denying activities in their stead. Substitutes can provide partial and temporary relief, but this decreases over time, and problems accumulate. Taking our problems out on others leaves us hungry and lost, separated from the very connections and relationships that can save us.

Evil is a thief with no power of its own. To feed off our energy, it goes where we keep our energy—in social relationships. Psychic illness attacks the very connections of life. It preys upon unmet human needs and drives and feeds off the energy released from damaging and breaking relationships. This is the oldest of schemes: look at the atom and the energy released when we pull it apart. Your digestive system breaks chemical bonds to extract energy from food. Physics, chemistry, and biology teach us that all metabolism works by creating and breaking bonds. Culture is no different. Our history is filled with the stories of people who rose to power by knitting together far-flung groups and others who stole power by sowing conflict and fomenting division, demolishing what others had created. Without this stolen energy, psychic illness cannot survive. It is a parasite.

Psychic illness drives people to metabolize others, temporarily feeding a privileged few while digesting the larger system. It obtains its energy by splitting things apart and breaking them down. It creates nothing. This is not sustainable. A society based on this will fall. It will turn itself into rubble and eventually kill all in contact with it. Evil is a sick substitute attempt to solve problems and meet needs by exploiting and hurting others. It fails to work and leaves us bent and broken while creating problems for others, driving the wheel around.

Evil is a perverted thwarting of life, an inferior substitute for life's affirmation. It is second best, a sham that can never be realized. Life builds things. Evil breaks and steals things. It can only exploit, harm, and destroy—bald evidence of parasitism. Whatever power it possesses is derivative. Evil can never be anything other than inferior to life, the thing it feeds on. Evil is life's shadow (Jung, 1995), feeding on all that is good. Evil is a virus, an acquired parasite that must suck its energy from the psyche because it has no power of its own. It is an empty fraud.

This raises the question, *does psychic illness ever coevolve to live in a symbiotic relationship with a host, providing equal or more benefit than cost?* Behavior-borne virus is a cruel master. It does not share power, and it will turn on you the second it becomes advantageous to do so. There is no doubt that some individuals in some instances can make some gains by exploiting others. It would be naive to believe otherwise. Exploitation is common in nature and humanity, so there must be some benefit. To answer this question, however, we need to look at the alternatives to exploitation. Nature evolved two basic schemes for relation: competition and cooperation. Both provide some benefits under some circumstances. Neither is good nor bad, and both are necessary for life. Yes, exploitation, a form of competition, can yield benefits. So can cooperation. So, the *real* question, the answer to the viability of evil, becomes, *how effective is exploitation relative to cooperation? How effective is theft relative to cooperative production?*

This brings us to the availability of disconnected and unexposed virgin populations. There are none. Human progress and globalization have knitted countless interdependencies into the fabric of human life. We have become joined together. As we connect our lives in ever more ways, cooperation becomes increasingly more beneficial than theft. My ongoing relationship with you will be far more profitable to me than my killing you and walking away with your wallet. This is the long game.

In nature, first contact can be difficult and competition fierce, but interdependencies are worked out to mutual advantage over time, and cooperation brings prosperity. You don't feed on your own kind. That would be suicidal. In this way, the system of life long ago moved from unicellular life to multicellular life, a type of systemic evolution, an emergent jump to a higher order of being. Jumps have happened many times in the past;[1] they always involve newfound connection and cooperation, and we are on the cusp of another one now. This is the current developmental stage of our planet, as humanity struggles to coalesce into a larger system more beneficial for all.

Reciprocation and cooperation benefit both individuals and groups. All major religions promote these and recognize them as essential to morality. Charles Darwin (1871/1930) saw human morality as rooted in social instincts that increase one's chances of survival. Reciprocation and cooperation have survival value. As highly social creatures, we humans are poorly served by strategies of exploitation and parasitism. Such strategies unnaturally enrich

---

[1] As discussed in Chapter One of *Psychic Illness* (Sweitzer, 2001 & manuscript in preparation), emergence produces a whole greater than the sum of its parts. Systems—including microorganisms, plants, forests, animals, muscles, brains, cultures, economies, weather, and the internet—are nested, emergent entities. Examples include elementary subatomic particles > composite subatomic particles > atoms > molecules > compound molecule > macromolecule > organelle > cell > tissue > organ > organ system > organism > population > community > ecosystem > biosphere. Other examples include cosmic dust > accretion cloud > celestial body > star system > star cluster > galaxy > galaxy cluster. Emergence involves dynamic, progressive transformation, and these examples are at various stages of emergence.

a few while impoverishing the remainder of the population. They are suboptimal.

Exploitation is not just wrong; it performs poorly. Cooperation is the better way. Cooperation makes better decisions and does a better job organizing labor, increasing productivity, distributing resources, reflecting true costs, allocating risks, decreasing conflict, ensuring safety, and increasing prosperity—all major issues facing us today. All pain cries out for attention and care. We will learn to cooperate for no other reason than if we don't, we will not survive. Our species will either emerge and jump to a higher order of being, or we will die. There are no other paths to survival. We are approaching the end of an age, and it is time to move forward and grow.

Proof #4: Evidence of Growth and Development

Everything that lives grows and develops. As organisms mature, they change size, shape, and function. Cultural transmission requires a prolonged period of early learning for the psyche to develop. There is much to learn and practice, and it must be relevant to the time and place the individual inhabits. During childhood, we are exposed to behaviors filled with information and instruction. To facilitate cultural transmission, we have open instincts to observe, imitate, practice, and learn the behaviors that we are exposed to. We grow and develop physically, intellectually, emotionally, socially, and morally, and when we reach maturity, we pass on what we have learned to others, starting the cycle anew. Cultural transmission is required for human growth and development.

Behavior-borne virus grows and develops as well, traversing a predictable life cycle through to maturity and reproduction. BBV gradually engages, invades, and plants itself in the psyche. It confuses perception, seizes control, imparts information and instruction, siphons resources, and induces pathological thinking and behavior. It infects us, grows and develops in us, and eventually matures and reaches the corruption phase, where it may reproduce by manipulating us to become self-defeating (controlled) or manipulative (controlling) when interacting with others.

BBV has identifiable developmental tasks. The receiver is engaged in a relationship. She acquires information and instruction: thoughts, behaviors, emotions, and beliefs. As BBV grows, she becomes confused and weakened and may eventually choose pathology over health. When this happens, she imitates, practices, and perfects the requisite skills. The cycle concludes with reproduction, the mature phase of psychic illness. Psychic illness requires highly specific and unnatural conditions to grow, develop, mature, and reproduce. These are all vulnerabilities that provide a wealth of opportunities to intervene and suppress it.

When unchecked, psychic illness is a progressive disease that can end in suicide, murder, or war. Adolf Hitler provides a case study of end-stage psychic illness. It devoured him, leaving a hollowed-out shell devoid of humanity. Too much money or power interferes with healthy development and feeds psychic illness by removing normal checks on our behavior. It is far better to have everyday stresses and reality-based constraints placed upon us. To develop properly and remain healthy, we need normal, everyday challenges—environmental press. These are good things. They keep us grounded, sharp, and strong. When children are not properly protected, cared for, loved, and socialized, when they do not face normal challenges, develop self-discipline and empathy, and when they possess too much or too little wealth or power as adults, they can become ill, and their behavior can become problematic for others.

To grow and develop properly, we need accurate feedback from our environment. The consequences of our actions provide valuable information and instruction that allows us to learn from experience and grow. Pleasure and pain—both physical and emotional—provide this feedback, telling us, "Do this ... don't do that." It's a guidance system. Reasonable limitations help us grow. Pain is valuable feedback necessary for survival. People born with congenital analgesia, the inability to feel pain, typically do not survive childhood due to injuries and unnoticed illness. Sometimes, pain is your friend. Normal checks on your behavior can make you strong and keep you aligned with the realities of your environment and the laws of life. Listen to what experience is telling you. Don't always wish for more. Wish for enough. Wish for a stop switch and gratitude, and you will do just fine.

Proof #5: Evidence of Adaptation

Living requires the ability to adapt, and adaptation is evidence of life. Viruses are the quick-change artists of biology, rapidly mutating to bypass established defenses and adapt to new conditions. Behavior-borne virus is a utilitarian opportunist. It does whatever works in a situation, whatever makes it more likely to survive. Like all cultural creations, BBV is supremely adaptable, changing as we change. This versatile adversary attacks with commando-like ruthlessness or the finesse of an artist, tailoring itself to the situation. In a changing environment, it finds and exploits new opportunities, adapting to the particular situation, culture, and psyche it inhabits and exploiting whatever resources and opportunities lay in its path. Psychic illness waxes and wanes, depending upon the nature of its surroundings and the host it inhabits. It manifests differently in different people, cultures, and situations.

Variation is necessary for adaptation as living organisms reach out to their environment, like tentacles probing for useful niches to inhabit and resources to extract. Psychic illness exhibits many forms and great variety. It manifests in such diverse activities as terrorism and teasing, racism and cattiness, murder and bullying. Its severity is determined by the virulence of our experience, the choices we make, and whatever opportunities BBV finds in its environment. A relatively mild expression of psychic illness is seen in the child who is roughed up by a bully and then "takes it out" (notice the literal meaning of this expression) on children or animals smaller than himself. More extreme manifestations are, thankfully, less common. The most severe cases involve depraved individuals driven to traumatize others, e.g., perpetrators of mass shootings and instigators of war.

Camouflage is an adaptation that can serve both defensive and offensive purposes. Evil grows in the dark, and psychic illness absolutely bristles with highly sophisticated forms of camouflage. It disguises its operations and hides from rational examination, for once its tactics are discovered and understood, its power is diminished. Psychic illness uses confusion for camouflage to avoid detection and conceal its actions and intentions. *Psychic Illness* (Sweitzer, 2001 & manuscript in preparation) devotes a chapter to this subject and describes forty-one strategies and tactics used by psychic illness to camouflage its operations.

Accommodation is a type of adaptation involving a single organism's transient adjustment in response to environmental changes. Eye focus and perspiration are accommodations. Psychic illness constantly assesses its situation and shifts tactics in response to changing conditions. It constantly probes the receiver for weaknesses and dynamically alters its strategies and tactics to accommodate them. The great variety of tactics used by psychic illness illustrates how it accommodates various situations. Accommodation is evidence of life.

Parasitism is a type of adaptation that requires a close, form-fitting, highly adapted relationship between parasite and host. A living organism, psychic illness is subject to the laws of evolution. It changes as we change. It evolves as we evolve, changing with the culture and psyche it inhabits. Psychic illness shadows our every move, an impression of darkness formed and defined by an absence of light. Parasitism is evidence of adaptation and life.

Rapidly adapting to and exploiting new technology, psychic illness penetrates, inhabits, and exploits modern media and networked computers. It also adapts to changed institutions and individuals. We now see new problematic behaviors that were not present in the past but have become common, illustrating the adaptation of psychic illness to changes of its environment. For example, some people now leave the news turned on in their homes throughout the day. This is not normal behavior, and it suggests subtle persuasion with addictive alteration of behavior. Doomscrolling, the obsessive urge to scroll through negative news, has become a problem, and we now read about "digital detox" and how to "break up" with your phone. These developments beg the question of who and what is controlling our minds, emotions, and behavior. BBV and psychic illness are highly adaptable and make ready use of changed environments and newly available technology. The prospects of what BBV might do with artificial intelligence and quantum computing are truly frightening.

Adaptive radiation occurs when environmental changes make new resources available, creating new opportunities to exploit and niches to fill. Species then diversify into new and different forms, and parasites may inhabit new types of hosts. BBV exhibits adaptive radiation. It assumes many forms and infects a variety of hosts and vectors. The forms it assumes and the vectors it inhabits are determined by the culture it occupies, the hosts and resources available to it, and the defenses it encounters. Like a thief casing a house, psychic illness systematically probes for vulnerabilities to exploit and resources to steal. BBV today is transmitted by a variety of hosts and vectors, more than in the past, and this variation and expansion is evidence of adaptive radiation, something only living things do.

BBV is highly opportunistic, exploiting whatever resources and opportunities it discovers in its environment. Psychic illness assumes many forms, from gossip to disinformation to child abuse to suicide bombing. These problems are so diverse that in the past, we overlooked their common elements and failed to recognize their similarities and universal operations: people exploiting and mistreating other people for illicit advantage and unwholesome gratification. These highly varied forms of psychic illness are evidence of adaptation. They are evidence of life and disease.

Proof #6: Evidence of Reproduction

Behavior-borne virus behaves predictably, transmits systematically, and reproduces reliably, making it vulnerable to the scientific methods we use against other infectious diseases. Psychic illness is transmitted through behavior, and behaviors define its life cycle. The process always begins with engagement and ends with corruption (when corruption is chosen). When not checked, BBV can persist over time, become a lifelong process, and it may eventually be passed to others, where it can begin the cycle anew. Listening to the stories of those affected reveals BBV's intergenerational nature: when it manages to survive, the virus can leave a generations-long chain of infected hosts. This stubborn persistence provides a facade of normalcy, which helps explain our mistaken belief that evil is an inevitable part of life. It is not. It is chronic infection by an external agent.

The steps and methods used by psychic illness frequently interconnect, with strategies and tactics often employing and supporting several others. They are interdependent, mutual catalysts that support and strengthen each other. These are links of a chain, ropes of a net, filaments of a web, all drawn together to form a single trap with a single purpose: domination, corruption, and control of the receiver.

The Psychic Illness Cycle

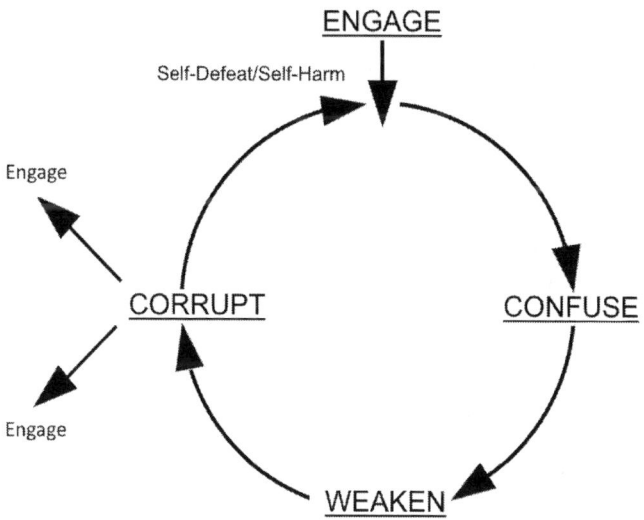

STEP 1: Present a problem.
  a. <u>Engage</u>: Psychic illness exploits existing problems, creates new problems, thwarts and blocks needs and drives, and prevents the natural, healthy resolution of problems. These are done to inflict pain, engage the receiver, and stimulate pathological activity for relief. For controlling receivers, engagement is accomplished more through preferential treatment, indulgence, vice, and providing opportunities to wield power over others.

STEP 2: Block resolution of the problem.
  b. <u>Confuse</u>: Transmitters say and do things to confuse the receiver. These tactics include various forms of stealth and camouflage to misrepresent situations, motives, and responsibilities.
  c. <u>Weaken</u>: Transmitters say and do things to weaken the receiver, reduce resistance, and make the receiver more malleable and receptive to pathological change.

Expended energy meant to resolve problems is diverted to destructive ends.

STEP 3: Encourage pathological problem-solving.
Pathological thoughts and behaviors are suggested and coerced, and opportunities are provided to encourage corrupt choices.

STEP 4: Choose corruption.
These actions are performed by the receiver-cum-transmitter. There are two corruption pathways.
d. <u>Transmit</u>: Controlling, exploiting, or harming others.
e. <u>Enable</u>: Allowing others to control, exploit, or harm you, or otherwise engaging in self-defeating or self-harming behavior.

When you see psychic illness naked and exposed like this, it looks vulnerable. It is vulnerable. You can see opportunities to interfere with its processes, disrupt its operations, and prevent its reproduction. Exposing psychic illness reveals the extent to which it depends upon stealth and subterfuge to operate. Its need to access new hosts to survive also makes BBV vulnerable. Psychic illness requires very specific and unnatural circumstances to operate, and these can be disrupted and often even eliminated.

We are not villains; we are hosts. Psychic illness infects and poisons us. It replaces our plans with its plans, pushes us to reenact our problems and infect others. Without our involvement, it cannot reproduce. It is one thing to subject a person to a difficult experience but quite another to get them to repeat it. Psychic illness engages us with manufactured problems, blocks their resolution, and encourages vices, addictions, and other substitutes that create similar issues for others to recruit them into the disease.

Reenacting old problems breathes new life into them. It is unfair to the people it uses, it creates similar issues for them, and it doesn't even work. You can't just dump your problems off on someone else by doing to others what was done to you. It doesn't work that way. Substitutes change nothing. Substitutes are a trap that suppresses symptoms, provides an illusion of improvement, and ends efforts for change. Substitutes keep us stuck. If you do not change and grow, the problems that you have now will be with you 50 years from now. We grow out of problems by facing and addressing them. As payment for our effort, we become stronger, more aware, and more effective. This is the better way.

Individuals do not invent psychopathology. They learn and choose it. Psychopathology is the predictable result of unhealthy environments, dysfunctional relationships, improper incentives, and bad choices. The transmitter is both damaged and damaging. There is a pattern to these acts, and where there is a pattern, there is information and meaning. Why is it that people who hurt others have so often seen harm and been harmed? Must we do to others what was done to us? Why is this a common precursor to psychopathology? Psychopathology is communicable. It reproduces through social behavior, and when we see something reproducing that we hadn't thought to be alive, red flags should go up and bells start ringing, alerting us to the presence of an undetected organism and compelling us to search for other life functions such as metabolism, activity, and growth. Psychopathology follows harm. Harm *causes* psychopathology. Stop the harm, and evil dies. Evil is frail. Evil can be stopped. We are more powerful than we know, and our oldest and worst enemy is exceedingly vulnerable.

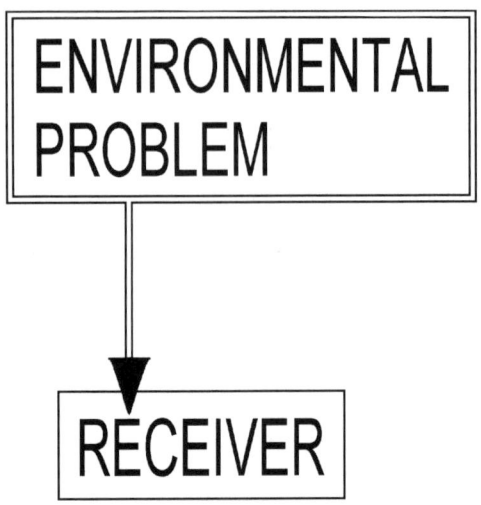

STEP 1: Present a Problem

The transmitter creates artificial problems, an unnatural environment crafted to engage the receiver through poor fit and conflict with his surroundings. These problems originate outside the receiver. They are forced upon him, invade his legitimate personal boundaries, and stimulate pathological activity for relief.

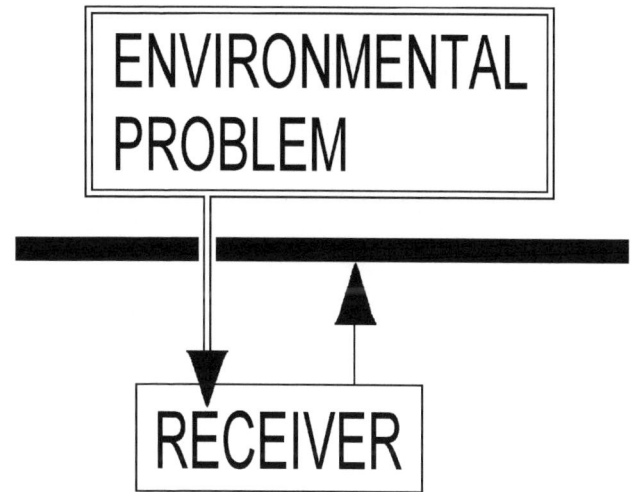

STEP 2: Block Resolution of Problem

The transmitter continues to create problems for the receiver and now also blocks efforts to address these problems. The receiver adapts to this situation by altering his behavior, thoughts, emotions, and beliefs. The arrow extending from the receiver represents where he believes his problems are located and where he focuses his efforts for change.

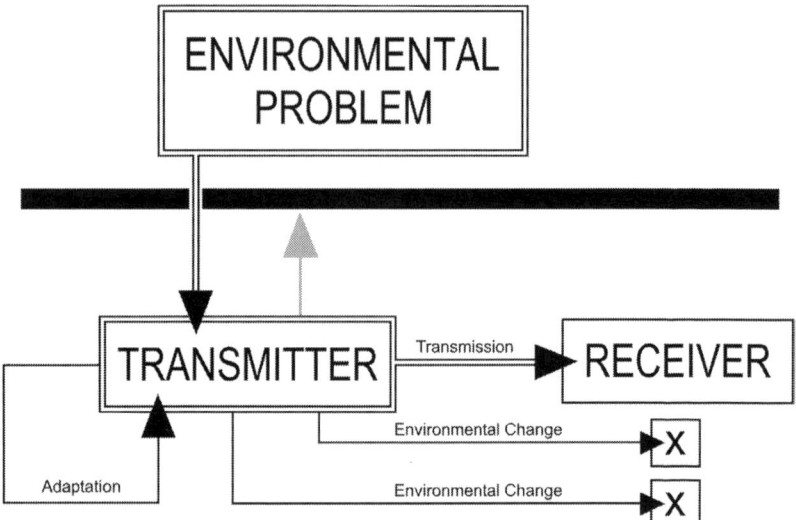

STEP 3: Encourage Pathological Problem-Solving

The receiver decreases and eventually abandons his efforts to directly address pathological problems in his environment. Continuing his search for relief, he refocuses his energies. He adapts by changing himself, others, or things in his environment that are not problems (X). In a misguided effort to relieve his problems, the receiver may now transmit or enable psychic illness.

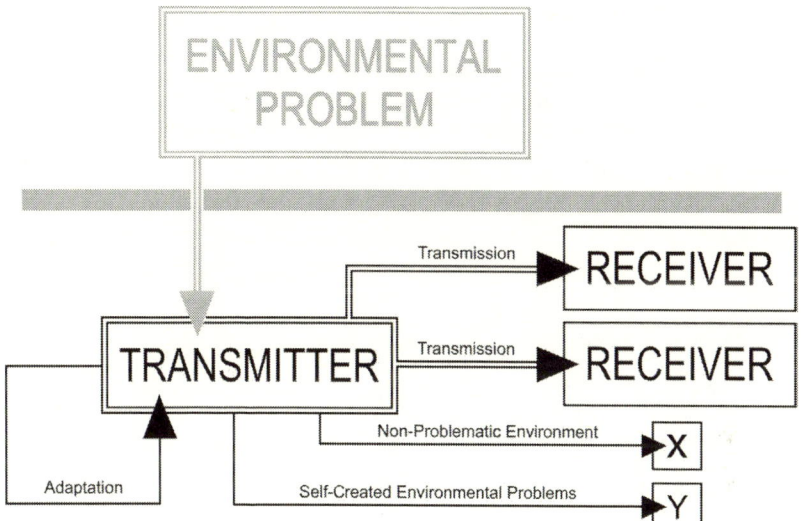

STEP 4: Choose Corruption

The environmental problem is now absent, or resolution is no longer blocked. This typically occurs following the receiver's emancipation from his family of origin. Internalized conflicts continue to press for psychic reorganization, driving the illness after the original problems no longer exist. The receiver now finds himself unable to adapt to a problem-free environment and change back. Activities adopted to cope with past circumstances continue, although they are no longer appropriate in present circumstances. What began as an environmental problem is now a self-perpetuated personal problem located inside the individual. The receiver's actions exert stress outward to his environment, creating issues for others similar to those he first experienced, completing the cycle. The former receiver has now become a transmitter.

Outward-directed energies focus on non-problematic parts of one's environment (x), creating or contributing to environmental problems (y), and transmission to a receiver or receivers. Inward-directed energies can include adaptation and (for a controlled person) self-defeating or self-destructive activity and allowing others to exploit or harm him. A receiver-turned-transmitter can also be described as a host, an organism in which another organism lives. Hosts can transmit to several new receivers and thereby greatly multiply the impact of the illness. Culpability begins when we participate in the psychic illness cycle, trying to solve our problems by exploiting or hurting others or allowing others to exploit or harm us.

~ ~ ~

Viruses exploit their host's resources to reproduce and complete their life cycle. It's a hack job. The common cold changes human behavior, compelling us to sniffle, cough, and sneeze to spread germs. Psychic illness also changes human behavior, compelling us to create problems that engage and infect people. The receiver may internalize unresolved problems (they become conflicts) and eventually seek unhealthy relief, creating similar issues for others that perpetuate the cycle. Psychically ill families repeat unhealthy behaviors that situational and biological factors cannot explain. Psychic illness may occur within any relationship, but it is most pronounced in parent-child relationships and between partners.

Individuals begin the cycle as passive receivers. If the disease succeeds, which is by no means certain, they will complete the psychic illness reproductive cycle by becoming transmitters, actively choosing and participating in the illness and creating problems for others to infect fresh recruits. Alternately, controlled people may complete the reproductive cycle by passively allowing others to control, exploit, or harm them, becoming self-defeating, or engaging in outright self-harm. This is a common strain of psychic illness, and self-defeating/controlled people are often seen in therapy. I have learned much from them.

Whichever form the virus assumes, controlled or controlling, corruption requires choice and participation. Choosing an illicit strategy, choosing to harm others instead of dealing with your own issues, is the essence of corruption. If you habitually take your problems out on others or let others harm you, reproduction is accomplished, and the psychic illness reproduction cycle is complete. There is, however, some good news here. We are contaminated not by what goes into us (our experiences, life events, or what happens to us) but by what comes out of us: the choices we make, how we respond to life events, what we think and do. Choose well.

For most infectious diseases, including psychic illness, prevention is more effective than healing. It is better never to face such a thing than to fight an infection. To survive, psychic illness must pass between generations, from older to younger people (vertical transmission). This occurs most often in parent-child relationships. Psychic illness is also passed horizontally between persons who are more-or-less equivalent in age to radiate out and spread across a population. Horizontal transmission can occur between siblings, partners, schoolchildren, neighbors, friends, co-workers, acquaintances, or even strangers. Psychic illness also reproduces on a larger scale by exploiting groups and institutions such as schools, work sites, news and entertainment media, corporations, political parties, and even governments. Psychic illness scales well and rapidly, and organized groups and institutions have committed some of history's worst deeds.

**HOSTS AND VECTORS
OF PSYCHIC ILLNESS**

1. The human psyche – e.g., thoughts, emotions, behaviors, and beliefs. Logic would suggest this was the original host.
2. Cultures – e.g., aberrant group practices, pathological (unhealthy and life-denying) myths, beliefs, prescriptions, proscriptions, and practices.
3. Subcultures – e.g., some online communities, outlaw gangs and clubs, extremist and terrorist groups, nationalist organizations, the criminal underworld, and organized crime.
4. Institutions – e.g., corrupt formal and informal practices of public and private institutions, legislatures, corporations, courts, codified laws, regulations, rules, and policies, political bodies, lobbying entities, law enforcement organizations, criminal justice systems, and news media dedicated to disseminating false and misleading information to manipulate public opinion, etc.
5. Families – e.g., manifested in child, sibling, partner, and elder exploitation and abuse and intergenerational trauma.
6. Media – e.g., the internet, broadcast news, printed text, photographs, film, social media, art, digitized media, and some pornography, etc.
7. Computers – e.g., viral computer code electronically transmitted and stored on a chip, disk, tape, optical media, and paper. Because computers and psyches each require the presence of a qualitatively different host in which to activate, they are infected by separate strains of psychic illness.

Proof #7: Evidence of Pandemic Spread: Going Viral

Given the right conditions, psychic illness spreads exponentially, reproducing vertically and horizontally. We have created optimum conditions for the spread of psychic illness, and single transmitters can now command audiences in the billions. Global media collect and report news of each day's worst deeds to us. Mass media, mass transportation, and mass culture allow the mass transmission of psychic illness. As cultural transmission expands, culturally transmitted disease expands. Like all organisms, BBV multiplies exponentially until checked by some external limitation, its own alterations of its environment eventually slowing its reproduction. We have removed many of these natural checks, allowing BBV to reproduce at unprecedented rates. Look around you now and observe the result.

New technologies make it easy to anonymously spread false information and immoral instruction. There's less filtering than in the past, fewer barriers to publication. Unlike traditional forms of media, the internet is decentralized and interactive, and content is relatively unmoderated. The potential for transmitting psychic illness is staggering. The world has suddenly been opened wide, and most individuals now have access to billions of other people. This is an epidemiological disaster.

For parasites, it is a bonanza. Old limits are gone, and the internet teems with pathological content. Mass communications, public broadcasting, and now the internet enable a single speaker to instantly transmit her ideas to countless others across the globe. Communications are no longer confined by geography or time.

Life has never done this before. The biological equivalent would be to enable a single organism to infect all present and future members of a species, regardless of time and place. Ideas and instructions now explode across cultures at speeds unknown in the natural world. New technologies have made cultural transmission far more powerful and us far more vulnerable. The consequences have been devastating.

In just a few generations, psychic illness has hollowed out America, changing us from a country where hundreds of thousands of boys laid down their lives to protect us from the fascist Nazi menace into a country flirting with fascism, where millions of people refused to wear a mask or get a jab to protect their neighbors and health care providers during a deadly pandemic. We are a shadow of what we were. The bad news is that cultures and brains can be hacked and manipulated for pernicious ends. The good news is that cultures evolve in response to psychic pathogens. Every culture has an immune system. Cultural transmission and cultural evolution produce not only viruses; they also produce antibodies.

In the past, the stories we told each other were moral lessons and cautionary tales. They had a protective effect. When I was a boy, the shows we watched were unequivocal: people who acted reasonably and treated each other well prospered. There was evil in the world, but you met it head-on, and what you stood for defined who you were. Standing up to evil made you stronger. It made life better. The bad guys got what they deserved, and evil did not pay. Today, in media and politics, poisoning minds has become a familiar business model. Delusional victimhood is actively encouraged, as is forcibly "taking back" whatever you imagine to be rightfully yours. The appeal is obvious: you are entitled to whatever you want. No effort, logic, or morals are required.

Poison. Facts, reality, and other people's rights—those pesky things that interfere with psychic illness—are no longer necessary considerations. People are told that reality is relative. You get to make up "alternative facts" and create your "own truth." Poison. Your rights are sacred, and if you feel it, then it must be true. Other people have no rights. Shows explore the depredation of the soul in morbid detail, and there is no path to salvation, healing, growth, or even learning. We have lost our way.

We have built our civilization upon the seven deadly sins. We celebrate greed, sloth, envy, lust, and gluttony and then proudly call ourselves exceptional while we angrily exploit each other and devour, depopulate, and wreck this planet. We are deluded, and it serves none but the virus.

Changes in how people and microbes interact create new avenues of infection. When people first settled in villages thousands of years ago, microorganisms more freely circulated in close quarters. There were more bodies nearby to infect and feed upon, and parasites and infectious diseases thrived. Today, the internet and social media place vast numbers of minds in close contact, freely communicating in relatively unmoderated forums, creating favorable conditions for the propagation of behavior-borne viruses. There has never been such easy access to so many psyches. There have never been so few barriers to twisting truth, bending minds, and stoking lower animal instincts. With so many brains to feed on and so few antibodies to interfere, the internet, as it exists today, is an ideal vector for psychic illness.

We have lost our way, misled down a dark path by this most treacherous foe. The past 20 years have seen a radical shift to extremist media that hype and exaggerate existing problems and fabricate fictional stories they "report" as problems to engage us in their psychopathology. Lacking facts to support their agenda, they just make stuff up. Their poison is crafted to feed biases, insecurity, prejudice, anger, and fear—the very worst of man. These concocted, manipulative lies (e.g., 9/11, birtherism, Pizzagate, the Big Lie, and other baseless conspiracy theories) generate advertising revenue, political contributions, influence, and political power that benefits a wealthy and powerful few at the expense of the many. Electronic media have proven alluring and persuasive in ways we did not anticipate, damaging our mental health. The media contribute to anxiety, addiction, sleep disturbance, eating disorders, mental disorders, social isolation, suicide, political polarization, radicalization, assault, and murder. Try to identify a single type of noxious thinking or behavior that is not actively fed by electronic media today. Moral and spiritual values protect us, but they are being replaced by self-righteous and self-serving poison that is antithetical to freedom and self-rule.

Misrepresentation is the heart of fraud. Psychic illness spins problems, defining them in a way that denies their existence, shifts blame, and excuses inaction. This strategy is now widely used in response to large-scale social, economic, and environmental problems. The appeal is obvious: you're off the hook. You can do whatever you want, and you get to blame others while you do it. Because such actions are not based on reality, ignored problems worsen until they become unavoidable. By then, your options have narrowed, and you are more stressed, desperate, and ready to compromise and serve the virus. *Social, economic, political, and environmental dysfunction and failure are part of the plan.* Dysfunction and failure create stress and pain, motivating disadvantageous compromises and unhealthy change. Stress breaks things down. Stress changes things. For the psychically ill, stress, pain, and problems are a good idea. They are useful tools for manipulating people. We now have politicians refusing to enact stricter laws to address the sale of firearms even though most Americans want this (Gallup, 2023), and mass shootings are occurring daily. Using culture to guide our actions only works when we are alert to problems and respond to them, when we are accountable and responsible, using foresight and intelligence to address problems and remove obstacles. Absent this, the virus can have its way with us.

Psychic illness can be largely removed from media while maintaining free speech. If you do not believe this, compare today's media content to that of half a century ago. Psychic illness has invaded and infected the media, making it increasingly manipulative, driven by profit and power to the exclusion of reason and morals. Poison words and poison pens poison minds. Each instance of bad behavior is efficiently collected, reported, and eagerly consumed. Our appetite for misdeeds seems limitless. The media poison us, and we lap it up. This is not healthy. Freedom of speech does not bestow a right to infect people. When an individual commits suicide, we understand that their mind contained unhealthy thoughts, emotions, and beliefs. Before our species commits suicide, we need to understand that our culture contains unhealthy thoughts, emotions, and beliefs.

I know addiction when I see it, and we sorely need an intervention. Just where do you think this is going? How do you think this will end? I feel like the brakeman on a runaway train headed for a cliff. I run down the aisle shouting and shaking people, but they do not awaken. It is a ghost train. We slumber under the narcotic of alien influence, poisoned by nightmares masquerading as reality. If we do not awaken and arrest this process, we'll all die.

There is nothing to be gained by my recounting here all the problems we now face. It has become painfully evident that the world is rapidly deteriorating. We are beset by a host of problems that are only getting worse with time. They are all tied together by a single, common thread of infectious misbehavior spun by the ultimate virus. If you seek evidence of the pandemic spread of psychic illness, look around you now. We are surrounded by it. We are steeped in it. We are permeated by it. Beware: the water is heating up.

Proof #8: Evidence of Defenses

Psychic illness uses an entire battery of sophisticated defenses that betray a sick genius for manipulating people while eluding conscious awareness. Impairing perception, weakening resistance, draining resources, and recruiting new hosts, this is no accident or mistake. This is infection.

Invading microbes slip past the defenses of their host. Infection is war, and psychic illness uses deception, subterfuge, and confusion for camouflage. It must hide from rational examination, for when its tactics are discovered and understood, they are weakened and become vulnerable to reason, conscience, and social sanction. All pathogens need a particular medium to inhabit and multiply. Some bacteria need a warm and moist place; others require the absence of light and oxygen. Biological viruses need DNA. Psychic illness hides inside the unconscious mind, safe from the checks of reason and logic. The unconscious mind is primitive, irrational, and emotional, containing powers and weaknesses all its own. To infect and endure, psychic illness must conceal its presence to avoid detection and awareness. It does this by exploiting the peculiar vulnerabilities of the psyche to confuse us.

Our brain is a complex system composed of many and varied parts, layered subsystems stacked from primitive to modern, evolved over hundreds of millions of years. The brain stem, the oldest and lowest part, controls physiological functions such as heartbeat and breathing. Further up and later in our brain's evolution is the reptilian complex (MacLean, 1990) which regulates aggression, ritual, territory, and social hierarchy. Above that lies the mammalian limbic system, responsible for emotions and social bonding. The cerebral cortex is the most recent part of our brain, crowning the more primitive parts below. The cerebral cortex is responsible for executive functions of reason, planning, intuition, self-monitoring, and critical analysis (Lezak, Howieson, & Loring, 2004).

There is a reptilian brain buried within the human brain. We're running Holocene software on Permian hardware and finding that some things are hard-wired. Psychic illness appeals to older, more primitive parts of the brain, enticing, seducing, and provoking us by engaging base instincts, appetites, and desires—to evade detection by the frontal lobe and consciousness. It may even use the frontal lobe's powers of rationalization and deception and leverage the mammalian limbic system's need for social connection to prosecute its ends.

Like any good criminal, psychic illness is careful to leave no evidence. It hides in darkness, avoiding exposure and examination to maintain control. Discovery weakens it. The receiver must not see his situation for what it is; he must not become aware of his world or himself within it. He learns to ignore his body, forget his thoughts, suppress his feelings, and abandon his beliefs. These faculties provide important clues to his circumstances, and it is unhealthy to deny them. If a controlled person asks too many questions and attempts to expose the pathology, she will be punished. If she persists, she will be ostracized to prevent her dangerous ideas from spreading to others.

Pathological instructions are subtly communicated to prevent their discovery and examination. Simultaneously transmitted through multiple senses and levels of awareness to different parts of the brain, the multichannel and multilevel commands of psychic illness conceal their presence, purpose, and contradictions. They escape detection and neutralization by the conscious mind. Psychic illness plays to our emotions to bypass consciousness, reason, and logic. It manipulates unconscious fears and insecurities and uses insinuation and implication to convey subtle threats. These messages contain hidden, illogical assumptions and some shreds of credibility that presuppose their demands are proper and made by appropriate persons. These tactics work the receiver like a marionette while hiding off-stage and out of sight. Limited only by the transmitter's creativity, they disguise their presence, divert attention from real issues, and drain valuable energy.

To conceal its presence and confuse us, psychic illness instills cognitive distortions such as emotional reasoning, labeling, overgeneralizing, polarized thinking, arbitrary inferences, catastrophizing, and mental filtering. Cognitive distortions restrain and control us. They engage irrational emotions to limit what we can perceive, learn, and feel, the relationships we can form, and the actions we can take. This is mind control.

Many acts of evil occur not as intentional, conscious decisions to harm others but as the result of an unquestioning, self-serving sense of being in the right. Or just not caring. People who insist they are right, regardless of all evidence to the contrary, who believe that their cause is just, no matter how many people they harm, have committed some of history's most horrible deeds. All that is required is a willful disconnection from reality, a refutation of other life, a voluntary blindness to the sanctity of all souls. This is self-delusion, the virus concealing its presence even from the infected. A lie is more effective when you believe it. The fanatic is so focused on his cause—how he defines it—that the broader picture, the evils he commits, passes unnoticed and dismissed. Or he uses mirror image lies to portray his cowardly acts as heroic deeds, a self-righteous "cleansing" of the evils he rightly senses are afoot in the world but mistakes their location.

Behavior-borne virus is a highly evolved and sophisticated organism with multiple infection and defense strategies. Like herpes, BBV uses stealth. It masquerades as appropriate thinking and behavior and hides in the unconscious mind, evading detection and neutralization by conscience and culture. Like rabies in dogs, BBV compels people to forcibly engage others. Like measles, BBV can go dormant and lay in wait for the right conditions to infect new persons. Like the common cold, BBV alters human behavior to facilitate its spread. Like HIV, BBV attacks and may even hide in immune functions of cultural values. Like COVID-19, BBV rapidly mutates, often faster than we can adapt to it.

Infectious organisms employ defenses to maintain their operations, evade detection, and prevent their neutralization and removal. The primary defenses of psychic illness are camouflage and stealth. Psychic illness conceals its presence, confuses people, and disguises its actions, nature, purpose, and effect. It plants itself in the unconscious mind, evades detection, seizes control, and uses sophisticated defenses to thwart its discovery, neutralization, and removal. Masquerading as appropriate thought and behavior, persons infected with psychic illness may feel entitled, justified, indignant, angry, and even morally superior as they exploit and abuse others and commit heinous acts. Normal, healthy relationships are reciprocal, and we should be wary of self-serving behavior that harms others.

Psychic illness constructs a facade of well-being to conceal hidden pathology and prevent its being checked by personal conscience and social sanction. Some cult leaders and terrorists deliberately adopt and modify established religion to hide their corrupt purpose beneath the stolen legitimacy of a mainstream faith from which they have greatly deviated. Stolen valor is a similar camouflage. These illusions plausibly explain the relevant facts, lending credibility to the appearance of normal behavior. To understand sick situations, we must sift through layers of pretense to determine their actual function.

Psychic illness creates spurious feedback to gaslight and confuse us. It impairs self-awareness and problem-solving to make actions ineffective and prevent escape. For controlling transmitters, it encourages externalizing defenses of blame, denial, projection, anger, control, and violence. It uses mirror-image lies, a form of projection that turns the truth inside-out, presenting a mirror image of reality. The transmitter essentially blames others for what he is doing. This is more than mere gall, for a bald-faced lie can be more believable than one that merely pieces facts together in a plausible fashion. Audacity lends credibility to a falsehood, especially when it is a mirror-image opposite of reality. The unconscious mind has difficulty distinguishing opposites and recognizing such lies, making distortions appear plausible when they reverse reality: war is peace, slavery is freedom, and ignorance is strength (Orwell, 1949/1987). For controlled persons, psychic illness encourages internalizing defenses of shame, inappropriate acceptance of responsibility, introjection, anxiety, and passivity.

> The actions of men are the best interpreters of their thoughts.
> —John Locke

To see what someone is about, look at their behavior. Ignore words. People lie with words. Lies are exposed by behavior. Behavior reveals what's inside a person, their thoughts, beliefs, and intentions. When speech quarrels with behavior, believe the behavior. Morality is measured not by what we say but by what we do, how we treat other people and other life. Peering beneath and stripping away the defenses of psychic illness makes it vulnerable and less effective. Without lies, it becomes much more difficult to do its dirty work.

Psychic illness uses prejudice not just to attack and exploit; prejudice also functions as a defense. Prejudice is a cognitive bias that distorts perception and creates habitat—safe places for BBV to live and hide. Prejudice causes us to respond to events and people in a manner that is not based on reality. This makes us less effective and creates injustice for others. The transmitter teaches a biased and pessimistic worldview: people are lazy and can't be trusted, and nice guys finish last. Other races, religions, nationalities, etc. (transmitters enjoy labeling people) are inferior. Prosocial behavior is a sign of weakness, evil is to be expected, and life is a merciless struggle for survival. He's got a bad attitude. Prejudice rationalizes unhealthy behavior and prevents escape. You cannot leave Hell when you are unaware that anyplace else exists.

Psychically ill people structure the world to conform to their expectations. Misinterpreting his environment, the transmitter responds inappropriately to people and events. Controlling persons create problems and injustice for others, while controlled persons can unconsciously create a world they at first only imagine and fear.

The lesson here is that reality is your friend. No purpose is served by seeing the world as any worse or better than it is. Distorted thinking is a major cause of mood disorders and behavior problems. Cognitive behavioral therapy teaches people to realistically evaluate and modify their thoughts and beliefs and correct cognitive distortions. The goal is to strengthen people by freeing them from unquestioned assumptions and beliefs, to help folks see the world as it is, choose effective strategies, work on what they can change, and accept or disengage from what they cannot. BBV is a coward and a bully, an empty fraud. It has only what power we give it, and we need not give it any power at all. Psychic illness hides from consciousness, vulnerable to its scrutiny and review. Caught between desire and scruples, consciousness is governed by the reality-oriented ego, the referee of the mind. Consciousness finds it unacceptable to attempt to solve our problems by hurting or exploiting others, so pathological activities are often hidden from consciousness as these sorts of gratifications are frequently unacceptable to the conscious mind. No one begins their life determined to harm another—it is unnatural to prey upon other members of one's species. But only part of our mind is occupied by consciousness. The lion's share sleeps down in the basement, working us like marionettes, invisible steel tethers occasionally glinting under a stray lamp and betraying their hold upon us. This shadowy realm operates not upon principles of reason and logic but raw emotion and primitive association. With courage, honesty, and humility, we can summon the strength to explore the hold of the mind and bring light to dark things that dwell within us.

Proof #9: Evidence of Offensive Strategies and Tactics

Carefully orchestrated, systematic, pathological acts repeatedly directed toward vulnerable people over time are the essence of psychic illness. This is personal terrorism, a series of organized, calculated, and traumatic assaults upon the psyche. Through elaborate behaviors, one person—often a parent or mate—trains another to interact with others in unhealthy ways that can continue even beyond the end of their relationship.

Infectious diseases shape human populations, history, and evolution. They change us; we change them. We coevolve. Pathogens stimulate immune responses, and we have evolved many sophisticated defenses against psychic illness. Evil has taught us about good. Psychic illness attacks these defenses because they threaten its survival.

Controlling transmitters seldom come to therapy unless they can use it for camouflage, often attending for no more than a session or two, dragged in by somebody else, and briefly making a show before beating a hasty exit. They aren't interested in changing or growing. They seek master-slave relationships where they can manipulate others into accommodating them. They are resource extractors who treat people like disposables. The offensive strategies and tactics of psychic illness are revealed through the behavior of persons infected by it.

<u>Controlling persons</u> use offensive strategies that:
1. Maximize (personal, political, economic, social, and physical) access, power, and control.
2. Maximize resource extraction and acquisition, e.g., emotional, social, physical, sexual, financial, political, economic, and military.
3. Maximize unwholesome gratification. This is typically accomplished through some combination of vice and controlling, exploitive, or harmful behavior.

4. Minimize the effort required to meet one's needs and address problems.
5. Minimize accountability and limitations on access, power, and control, e.g., mores, laws, moral standards, and institutional responsiveness to the public will.

<u>Controlled people</u> use defensive strategies that:
1. Use passive behavior to avoid conflict and disapproval and please others—to disarm aggression and provide a feeling of control.
2. Focus on others' needs and engage in pacifying and distracting activities, including self-neglect, self-depletion, self-defeating behavior, and self-harm.

These strategies are accomplished through cognitive and behavioral tactics that are readily described and quantified, making them amenable to scientific investigation and intervention. Pathological behaviors are most visible during transmission, a time of heightened pathological activity that puts the offensive methods of psychic illness on full display. Some of these methods were mentioned above; others are discussed below. *Psychic Illness: The Rise and Fall of Evil on Earth* provides a catalog of 171 existing strategies and tactics employed by psychic illness, as they often occur within the psychic illness cycle, with more or less success. Psychic illness uses four basic types of tactics to advance its life cycle: engage, confuse, weaken, and corrupt.

Engagement tactics are designed to establish and maintain a lasting relationship with the transmitter that is difficult to terminate. This relationship may be internalized and last long past the time of their interaction. In this way, the impact of the relationship can survive even the transmitter's death. Transmitters want to get inside the receiver's head, occupy their thoughts, perturb their emotions, and alter their behavior. This is typically accomplished by exploiting existing problems and creating new problems. For example, fishhook strategies involve problems that are easy to enter but difficult to escape. Engagement tactics may be crude and obvious, e.g., physical assault, or more sophisticated and subtle, e.g., multichannel communications using words contradicted by some combination of body language, tone, or behavior. Chapter Three of *Psychic Illness* describes 30 common engagement tactics.

Confusion tactics misrepresent circumstances, facts, behaviors, intentions, thoughts, situations, and relationships. They do this to avoid detection, bypass defenses, and prevent assistance or intervention by third parties. Confusion prevents the receiver from identifying the source of her problems and solving them. If you don't know where a problem exists (e.g., in yourself or your environment), you cannot effectively address it. Misdirected energies for change are not only ineffective; they also drain resources and create additional problems, further weakening her. Confusion tactics include lies, gaslighting, disguised communications, disabling of thought and emotions, impairment of perception, misrepresentation, misdirection, blaming, distortion of responsibility, etc. Chapter Four of *Psychic Illness* describes 44 confusion tactics.

Weakening tactics stress the receiver, isolate him from potential sources of support, thwart his efforts to resolve problems, reduce his resistance, squander his energies, extract his resources, and make him more tractable and willing to experiment with pathological strategies for addressing his problems. Stress facilitates change, and stressing individuals to threaten, weaken, depress, and alter them is a common feature of weakening tactics. These include depressing, threatening, neglecting, depriving, dehumanizing, kneecapping, demonizing, invalidation, indulging, frustrating, isolating, and shaming. Chapter Five of *Psychic Illness* describes 71 weakening tactics used by psychic illness.

Corruption tactics encourage pathological problem-solving. There are two corruption pathways. The first corruption pathway is to exploit or harm others. We say that a person "took it out on others" to describe this pathway. The second corruption pathway is to allow others to exploit or harm you, engaging in self-defeating behavior or active self-harm. The first pathway completes the life cycle by creating new transmitters. The second pathway rewards transmission, creates opportunities for developing transmitters to practice and perfect their transmitting skills, provides emotional pain for transmitters to feed upon, validates transmitters' worldview, provides a steady supply of resources for transmitters, disables guardians of vulnerable persons, and models psychopathology to children. Both pathways are pathological and further the reproduction of psychic illness. Chapter Six of *Psychic Illness* describes 26 corruption tactics.

Back Doors to the Brain

A back door to a computer is "An undocumented way of gaining access to a computer system. A backdoor is a potential security risk" (National Institute of Standards and Technology, 2023).

Back doors provide a means of gaining illicit access and control. Biological viruses use a bogus molecular key that disguises them as legitimate, permitting cellular access via a corresponding molecular lock on receptor sites of host cells. In a similar fashion, psychic illness exploits back doors to the brain to gain access to our minds. This is evidence of its offensive strategies and tactics and stealthy defenses. Some of these are briefly described below. For additional information, see *Psychic Illness* (Sweitzer, 2001 & manuscript in preparation).

Multilevel communications send inconsistent and contradictory information and instruction through different levels of awareness (e.g., conscious and unconscious) to conceal their contradictions and lack of validity from consciousness.

Multichannel communications are sent and received at different times through different sensory modes, e.g., speech and behavior, to conceal their contradictions and lack of validity from consciousness.

Protolanguage. The universal language of the unconscious mind and our first dialect, Protolanguage is used simultaneously with other more formal, modern, and conscious languages to enhance our powers of communication. Instead of words, Protolanguage uses nonverbal communication and sounds communicated outside the formal rules of speech and is frequently unconscious. Protolanguage is so old that many of its signals are shared with and understood by other animals, especially mammals and primates (Graham, 2023 #125). The word Protolanguage is used here as a proper noun, distinguished from the common noun protolanguage, which identifies one language as the precursor of another.

Primitive negative emotions. Provoking primitive negative emotions, e.g., insecurity, fear, anger, and outrage, can activate primitive brain circuits that override more modern faculties of reason and logic.

Addiction. Drugging prey is an old trick to confuse, weaken, and make one more pliable. Psychic illness typically initiates this by causing distress; childhood trauma is highly correlated with addiction (Maté, 2018). Addictions are about distraction, an attention shift to avoid pain and problems that eventually creates even more. Psychoactive substances alter judgment and decrease inhibition, and they can initiate a cycle of increasing distress, weakness, and desperation, preparing people for pathological changes in thinking and behavior. Progressive loss of control, characteristic of addictions, transfers control to the virus. Armies of chemically enslaved addicts pass money up the chain to their drug lords. When you see a cultural construction seizing control and stealing resources, think BBV.

Frustration. When our needs are not met in healthy ways, they can be transformed into weapons of destruction and used against us. Unmet needs do not diminish. They become stronger over time, and they can betray us. The transmitter frustrates and thwarts the receiver's needs and drives to engage and weaken him.

Indulgence. There is nothing wrong with occasionally indulging a person, but repeated indulgences become expected; people begin to feel entitled and adjust their actions accordingly. Excessive indulgence spoils and weakens a child. Things come too easy. Unchallenged, he does not push himself, develop his abilities, or grow. He remains weak and dependent, unable to address problems or fend for himself. He learns that gratification lies outside himself and learns to manipulate others to meet his needs and gratify his desires. He does not develop normal empathy. Indulgence also encourages vice, which also has a weakening effect.

Grievance thinking and rumination. Malcontent involves ruminative focus on perceived wrongs and blaming others for one's problems regardless of facts. Irrational grievances organize thinking, excuse failure, and explain one's dissatisfactions in a way that encourages aggressive and gratifying acting out while fantasizing that you are a righteous victim. In contrast, legitimate and rational grievances result from injustice and are not typically expressed aggressively or violently.

Stress. Stress is transformative. It changes things. It makes objects and people more malleable and easier to alter. Psychic illness uses stress strategically to weaken people, reduce resistance, and increase our willingness to change.

Depression. Depressed mood, feelings of powerlessness, helplessness, and hopelessness increase vulnerability and facilitate transmission. Almost any negative thought, emotion, or experience can be used to serve psychic illness. For this reason, transmitters apply stress to individuals to induce depression and weaken people's will and resistance.

Culturally embedded systemic incentives for advantage, wealth, and power. Perverse institutional incentives create inequality and poverty that feed and perpetuate psychic illness. Corrupt and rigged economies, political institutions, and social systems reward antisocial behavior. They are systemic pathology that is often transparent to those who benefit from it. Corruption begets corruption, making it easier for slippery people to work the system until it serves none but the slippery. For these reasons, political, economic, and social justice are imperative to prevent and heal psychic illness.

Stories. Stories are cultural tools that we have used for tens of thousands of years to coordinate the actions of large numbers of people over many generations (Harari, 2015). Stories can encompass all parts of the psychic illness cycle. They can effectively engage people, communicate a false narrative to confuse them, prompt pathological changes in thinking and behavior, and instill emotional beliefs that resist reason and logic. The stories used by psychic illness are simplistic sticky ideas—catchy, titillating, and self-serving tales that spin reality and play to prejudices to manipulate thoughts, emotions, beliefs, and behavior. Effortless to assimilate, they are most effective with people who do not practice critical thinking.

Lack of empathy. People who lack empathy are unbound by moral or ethical constraints, making them more easily influenced by psychic illness and more likely to commit evil acts. Empathy is developed through the experience of social connection and personal difficulty. People who have been indulged and spoiled, have not experienced healthy relationships, have not been taught empathy, or have been protected from life's normal challenges are at increased risk of becoming exploitative and abusive.

Instant gratification. Effortless and amoral strategies can provide instant rewards, but their costs are often hidden, deferred, and passed on to others. This can make effortless and amoral strategies addictive.

Sex. Emotional and sexual instincts attract and bond couples. Psychic illness turns sex into seduction, bait for a trap, and transmission can be played out in destructive sexual games. It is no wonder that evil often manifests in sexual behavior. Sexual desire can override reason and logic and be hijacked by psychic illness. This use of sex for alternate, unnatural, and pathological purposes betrays evil as a parasite. Any power that it possesses has been stolen from its host.

Need for attachment. We are social animals wired for attachment, and psychic illness exploits these instinctual ties. It abuses partnership, friendship, parenthood, dedication, commitment, and loyalty—anything that can attract, hold, and control. It turns these bonds into weapons of destruction to be used against us.

Base emotions. Transmitters manipulate and appeal to base emotions, such as insecurity, fear, anger, disgust, outrage, and greed. The transmitter provokes these emotions to defeat the checks of reason and logic and lure people into pathological thinking and behavior.

Vice. Vice (e.g., lust, greed, sloth, envy, gluttony, avarice, aggression, power, exploitation, abuse, and status) appeals to primitive and base drives while subverting higher human sentiments. All forms of vice involve gratification that, over time, weakens the receiver and makes him more easily controlled.

The unconscious mind. Evil often hides in the unconscious mind, where it can evade detection, examination, and neutralization by reason, conscience, and culture. The unconscious mind can conceal psychopathology from awareness, especially when it is self-serving.

This is evil's toolkit, offensive strategies and tactics to hack the brain. These access points are poorly defended and relatively unscreened by consciousness, making them effective channels for psychopathology. Psychic illness uses these to alter thoughts and emotions, bypass reason and logic, and manipulate us into accepting bad deals.

Proof #10: Evidence of Weaponization

Behavior-borne viruses have long been used to change minds, emotions, behavior, and beliefs; to gain advantage, seize control, win contests, take down opponents, and plunder resources. This is what parasites do. Racism provides an example of weaponized BBV. Racism is a myth that claims some persons, identified by their appearance, are inferior to others. This myth is weaponized to divide and harm people, extract resources, and advance some individuals over others. The lie of racism illustrates various aspects of weaponized BBV:

1. Subterfuge – Racism uses lies as a pretext to conceal the actual purpose and function of communications.
2. Propagation – Racism uses lies that disproportionately advantage some persons over others, including privilege and monetization, to encourage their dissemination by the people they advance.
3. Metabolism – Racism divides, harms, disempowers, and exploits to cause suffering and extract resources.
4. Intangibility – Racism is a weaponized cultural creation transmitted by behavior.

Propaganda and disinformation provide further examples of weaponized BBV, used for thousands of years to alter people's thinking and behavior. During World War II, Japan broadcast music and dispiriting misinformation—bait and poison—read by "Tokyo Rose" to damage Allied troop morale. State-sponsored Russian hacking operations spew a steady supply of disinformation into the United States to influence elections. A pro-People's Republic of China (PRC) network used online accounts to exploit U.S. COVID-19 divisions and peddle disinformation about a supposed U.S. origin of the virus (Serabian, R., & Foster, L., 2022). Iran used disinformation to exploit divisions and sow anti-Semitic discord among U.S. troops (Time, 2021). On January 6, 2021, a violent insurrectionist mob, fed fomenting disinformation, attacked and invaded the United States Capital (117th Congress Second Session, House Report 117-000, 2022). People were fooled into attacking their elected government based on the lies of propaganda. Propaganda and disinformation are evidence of weaponized BBV.

Behavior-borne viruses have been used throughout history to take down all manner of groups and individuals. Hitler needed the Jews, Stalin the disloyal, McCarthy the communists, Mao the counterrevolutionaries, and Pol Pot the intellectuals. All scapegoats, all used to gain and hold power. We are in an escalating information war, and the virus is eating our lunch. This enemy is not external. The enemy is within, and missiles, nukes, jets, and tanks are impotent against behavior-borne viruses. We must pivot our defenses and respond more effectively to the weaponization of psychic illness.

When we understand how psychic illness operates, we see that many human problems are not separate issues. They are related, a single malady expressed in various forms while retaining a common, critical thread: people mistreating other people. This is not natural, and despite what the virus would have you believe, it is not necessary. In nature, only an aberrance causes a creature to prey upon other members of its species. In humans, only psychic illness. These are not accidents. They are highly organized, weaponized tools of exploitation that occur regularly, systematically, and predictably. They can be stopped, healed, and prevented. We need to focus not just on individuals who act undesirably but also on the conditions that foster such behavior.

Psychic illness adapts to exploit whatever opportunities and resources it finds available in its environment. We don't have hate, homelessness, addiction, violence, and mental health epidemics; we have a pandemic of bad thinking and bad behavior. People are manipulated into controlling and self-defeating behavior by engaging their emotions and altering their thoughts. Division and discord are profitable. Dysfunction, fear, anger, and violence sell. For the corrupt, this is a business opportunity. Psychic illness has been monetized. It occurs between individuals and simultaneously on a much larger scale as corrupt influencers commandeer media, inject lies and confusion, weaken populations, and corrupt minds en masse. This extraction tool has been used against us for ages without our understanding what it is or how it works. Harnessing the enormous power of culture and impossible to control due to its habit of turning on those who wield it, psychic illness is the most dangerous weapon ever created.

Baseless Conspiracy Theories

We are losing people to toxic cocktails of titillating and outlandish conspiracy theories fed without reason or shame. Baseless conspiracy theories are crafted to distract attention, distort reality, provoke fear and anger, invite retelling, and, in the extreme, incite aggression. A form of mind control, baseless conspiracy theories are projections that accuse others of conspiracy, . They are distracting mirror-image lies designed to advance psychic illness. Baseless conspiracy theories seduce people into believing that they are privy to special knowledge and possess a superior understanding of invisible mischief underfoot in the world that eludes ordinary people. These beliefs—a mixture of overconfidence (Light, Fernbach et al., 2022), arrogance, grandiosity, and paranoia—serve to explain the world, maintain one's self-image (Douglas, Sutton, et al., 2017), and provide validation and membership. This can make people impervious to reason and consequences and believe absurd things while citing lack of evidence as proof of concealed wrongdoing—a self-reinforcing delusion.

Baseless conspiracy theories require no effort or evidence. They are easy. You get to make up and believe whatever you want, including that you belong to a morally superior, select, and privileged intelligentsia involved in a historic and noble cause that places you above the law. These emotionally appealing fantasies bypass the prefrontal cortex (responsible for reason, impulse control, and morality) and activate primitive circuits of tribalism and aggression. They are easily passed from one person to another through unguarded channels. These qualities can make conspiratorial thinking extremely dangerous, and persons infected with such thoughts can indulge in virus-driven inhuman behavior. Baseless conspiracy theories vandalize a culture, and history is filled with this kind of venom. We know how it ends. It ends in an orgy of evil. Truth, discoverable by facts, reason, and testable explanations and predictions, is the better way to walk through this world.

The Real Conspiracy

> Our democracy is in danger. The conspiracy to thwart the will of the people is not over ... January 6 and the lies that led to insurrection have put two-and-a-half centuries of constitutional democracy at risk.
>
> —Rep. Bennie Thompson

A genuine conspiracy now exists to overthrow governments and replace civilization with barbarism, to break apart all that is good and true and free in the world, feed off the remains, and torment the survivors. We've been down that path before, and it never ends well. The current situations in China, Iran, North Korea, and Russia provide cautionary tales. Humans are highly social animals, and cooperation has always been key to our survival. One of the reasons we so greatly developed social behavior was to defend against predators by banding together. Psychic illness seeks to destroy the social compact and divide us because social cohesion protects us from predation. Psychic illness attempts to strip our defenses and make us vulnerable so it can feed on us unimpeded. Fortunately, there are effective strategies to heal and prevent this.

Chapter 3

HEALING

An evil discovered is half healed.

—Jane Frances de Chantal

This chapter summarizes the strategies that individuals can use to heal from psychic illness. These methods are discussed in greater depth in Chapter Seven, *Healing*, found in *Psychic Illness: The Rise and Fall of Evil on Earth* (Sweitzer, 2001 & manuscript in preparation).

Become Aware of the Past in the Present. Past problems can intrude on the present without our being aware of them. These are opportunities to grow. If you repeatedly encounter the same sorts of problems, ask yourself why. Do you contribute to them? Where did you learn to act this way? Does this still work for you? When old problems step into your awareness and cause you pain, your unconscious mind has determined that you are ready to address them. Listen to your pain. Learn from it. Respond to it. Rework old problems in new ways. Grow. Many problems are healed in stages. You may have thought you were over them and not understand why they have appeared again, but this is normal. Take them off the shelf, work on them for a while, and put them back when you've sufficiently reworked them. Become aware of the past in the present and chip away at old problems.

Believe that Change is Possible. To move forward, we need hope, a realistic sense that things can be better. Without hope, there will be no effort, change, or growth. Without hope, we are stuck (Abramson, Metalsky, & Alloy, 1989). Hope frees us and opens the world wide. Hope and faith are exalting bridges that transform us from mere mortals to creatures able to reach beyond our circumstances. Hope is necessary for change, and a leap of faith takes us to new ground. Faith is belief in the unrealized potential of life, a commitment to values that gives meaning, defines who we are, and increases our abilities.

Choose to Change. We are determined less by what happens to us than by how we respond to it, what we think and do. We always have choice. Healing comes through awareness, choice, and effort. It comes through growth. To change, you must want to change, believe you can change, and act to bring it about. How much life will you let this thing squeeze out of you? How much pain must you endure? Change does not come easy, and healing is hard work.

Healing Psychic Illness

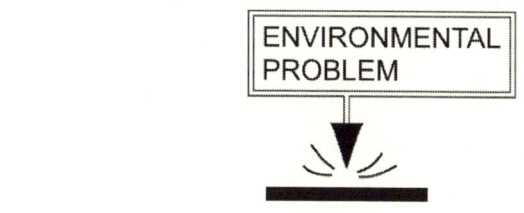

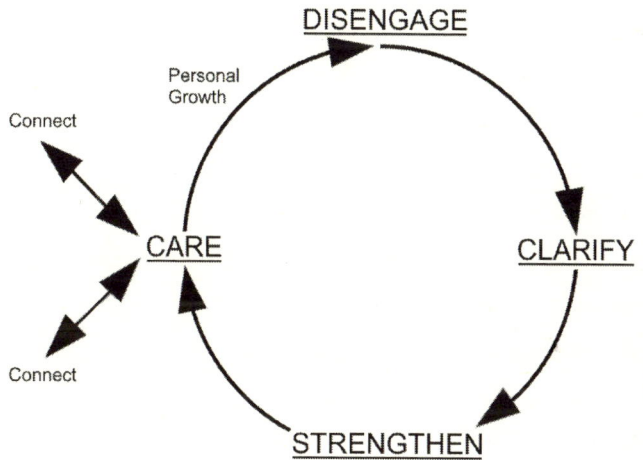

Disengage from Psychic Illness. Mahatma Gandhi and Martin Luther King Jr. demonstrated the awesome power of refusing to engage with evil, transforming the lives of millions of people with little more than character, determination, and justice in their armament. It is not enough to return hurt for hurt, for revenge never ends. To stop the cycle, we must let go of psychic illness. We must forgo revenge, refuse to be hurt, refuse to hurt others, and refuse to tolerate the hurting of others. The hurting must stop. Beware of people who encourage anger and fear. Limit your exposure to unhealthy influences and disengage from psychic illness.

Refocus Attention. Ask three people to describe an event each has witnessed, and you will receive three different reports. Attention alters perception and experience. We find what we look for. We *make* what we look for. Turn your mind from old harms. Stop gawking at unhealthy stories; this is dangerous entertainment. Do you eat rotten food? Of course not. It would make you sick. Be cautious about what media you consume, what you put into your mind, what you let live there, the stories you tell yourself. Look for beauty and kindness, and you will find them. Your world becomes what you look for and focus on.

Acknowledge Participation. We play a role in this illness, and owning this helps us stop feeding it and end it. To escape the psychic illness cycle, see your humanity, acknowledge your capacity to do to others what was done to you, and then choose other things. Face your dark side, observe how little it has to offer, and nurture yourself back to health. The ghosts of your past are dead and gone. It's you that you've got to live with. Come to terms with your past, build a new present, and work toward a better future.

Avoid Judgment. We blame others to distance ourselves from their evil acts, only to find ourselves bound more tightly to them. Judgment sets us apart and proclaims us beyond evil, but none of us are immune. We are caught in the middle: part good, part bad, striving to be something else. Judgment traps us in the psychic illness cycle. It implies that we are incapable of such wrongs, and denying our capacity for harm blinds us to our vulnerability and potential for wrongdoing. Only by recognizing the choices before us and admitting our ability to harm can we avoid doing to others what was done to us. Judgment interferes with compassion, forgiveness, and resolution. There is no avoiding the problems of this world, and the only way past them is through them.[2] Pain may not leave us untouched, but it need not destroy us. We can engage it, wrestle and grow with it, and move beyond it.

It is best to avoid judgment, but we do have responsibilities to protect each other and interfere with evil. When we see someone who is not resisting the virus, who has given themselves over to it while actively exploiting or abusing, the wrongful behavior needs to be called out and stopped. To prevent becoming contaminated, our motivation for taking action in such circumstances should be more to protect the innocent rather than to punish the wrongdoer. It is also imperative to disincentivize wrongful behavior throughout society, and this is an essential component of healthy cultures and institutions. Love, prevention, and protection are superior to anger, punishment, and vengeance.

Let Go of the Past and Get on with Your Future. Anger at injustice keeps us engaged and interferes with our moving on. To avoid doing to others what was done to us, we must recognize that

---

[2] Different situations call for different strategies. When you encounter the artificial and contrived problems of psychic illness, it is best to disengage from them and walk away when this is possible. This helps protect you from psychic illness. When you encounter life's natural problems or problems that result from your own actions, it is best to engage these and wrestle with them. This makes you stronger, more effective, and less likely to encounter or struggle with such problems in the future.

this is possible. We are more than transmitters or receivers. We are vectors and hosts, stuck inside the cycle, and our way out is to fill our lives with better things. Forgiving is not forgetting or condoning. It is letting go and bringing better things into your life. We overcome evil by acknowledging its potential to take root in ourselves and then choosing to grow other things.

Break the Chain. To protect ourselves from evil, we must be careful not to become too much like it. Your best weapon against evil is your heart, not your hardness, your compassion, not your outrage. Evil feeds on pride, anger, and fear. To carry these battles, you must develop strategies of your own, press the cause of life, and refuse to pass on your pain. Where the transmitter fought with guile, return honesty. Rise up and meet your circumstance. Trust in goodness and let love guide you to it. You are stronger than you imagine, and the world is more beautiful than you dream. This is a contest for posterity. Breaking the chains of psychic illness is noble work that allows life to be lived as it is meant.

Change Your Actions. With any kind of honesty, we eventually learn that no matter how we were hurt, we have become part of the problem. Explore your role in these difficulties. Change your behavior, thoughts, emotions, and beliefs. Responsibility brings growth, and what we do creates who we become. Activity shapes being. Change your actions, and you change yourself. Relationships are interactive. Change yourself, and you change the world.

Move On. Psychic illness requires sick situations, environmental press. If your environment is unhealthy, then change it or get out. If you can do neither, make your actions as healthy as possible and look for opportunities to leave. Let it go. Focus on things that help you grow, not artificial dilemmas that distract you, cause rumination, and squander your energy. Respond appropriately to problems: You cannot talk, think, or emote yourself out of situations you behaved your way into. Refuse to participate in sickness. Look for opportunities to change it and leave it. Do not adapt to it. Although the problems of psychic illness begin outside us, we may internalize them and do unhealthy things beyond the time required by our environment. If you are contributing to your problems, this is an opportunity to address them. What you learned can be unlearned and replaced with new learning. There is goodness in the world, and you are a living, breathing creature able to change and grow.

Deal with Real Problems, Not Substitutes. To make the most of life, see problems clearly and accept responsibility for your actions. Whose problems are these? Avoid blame and shame. Your goal is to address and resolve problems, not dodge them or pass them off on someone else. If these problems are your doing—things you could foresee and control—address them. If they are someone else's doing, deal with them. Don't avoid problems; pursue them. These are opportunities to grow. Work at correctly owning and disowning problems. Dispassionately examine your troubles and ensure that you address actual problems, not bogus distractions. Don't waste time on substitutes. You want to pull this thing out by the roots, not prune its leaves. What about problems that you cannot resolve? If there is no moral issue involved, walk away when you can. Disengage. Pick your battles wisely, and practice making healthy decisions. Take reasonable risks. Try new strategies, observe their results, and learn.

Make Emotions Work for You. Emotional pain is not the problem. Pain is a messenger, a signal filled with information and instruction. Pain alerts us to problems and motivates us to do something about them. Listen to your pain. Learn from it. What is it telling you? Why this signal? Why now? Negative emotions and challenging situations—pain and problems—are opportunities, signs that change will improve your life. These are chances to grow. Use the pain of problems, the results of not living well, to provide direction and motivate change. The pain that made you sick can now be used as it was meant—to guide you and propel needed change. Try different strategies. Use your distress to focus your efforts where they belong, where change is truly needed.

Exercise. When you are chronically stressed and physically inactive, your brain and body struggle under inappropriate levels of stress hormones and neurotransmitters. Chronic stress releases stress hormones that, over time, can become neurotoxic and alter your brain's structure and function (Perry, 2001). Your heart, liver, lungs, bowel, and other organs and systems can also be damaged as well. The brain is a master organ that controls the functioning of all other organs. Mind and body are connected. Work one, and you work the other. Your psyche is a system composed of parts, and when things go down, it's a network event. Your entire body is affected by stress, and effective health practices address both body and brain.

Cardiovascular exercise increases the metabolism of adrenaline and cortisol, reducing these stress hormones in your bloodstream and restoring a sense of personal control and calm. It also increases dopamine, endorphins, and serotonin, which can improve mood.

Play and recreation promote healing and resilience. Exercise, diet, and sleep are recognized causes of and treatments for depression. Physical activity stimulates the growth of new nerve cells in your brain, increasing mental activity and efficiency (Gage, 2003.) Find physical outlets for pent-up thoughts and emotions. Get your heart rate up. Cardiovascular exercise is a fast and effective way to boost psychic health. Walking is beneficial for mood and thinking as well. Bones, stomach, joints, lungs, heart, brain: every organ works better when we are active. Physical activity promotes relaxation, enhances sleep, clarifies thought, improves learning, and increases self-esteem. It changes how you view the world, how you feel about yourself, and your ability to take control of your life. Exercise is good medicine.

Cultivate Awareness and Understanding. Evil hides in darkness because light kills it. Live in the light. Strive to understand your history and label the things done to you to decrease their power. Be courageous. Ask questions and open yourself to new experiences. Face the harm done to you, to those who harmed you, and what you could do to others if you don't resolve these problems. Psychic illness needs confusion to operate, so don't be confused. Clarify. Cultivate awareness and understanding. When you seek a better way, your path will find you and make itself known.

You can only change what you see. Examine your actions and ask how they contribute to your problems. Watch how you interact with others, how they perceive you, and how you shape each other. Recognize that psychic illness meets some of your needs, and then ask what it does for you. Is this how you want to live? Is this all that life has to offer? Find a better way.

Respond to Your Preferences and Meet Your Needs. Evil feeds on unmet needs. Unmet needs weaken us and make us needy and vulnerable. Stop starving yourself. Your senses have not lied. You are hungry for a reason. Listen to your hunger. Learn from it. These are not the teasings of psychic illness; life delivers. Evil becomes unnecessary when we meet our needs, so nurture and feed yourself. Connect with people, places, and things that make you feel alive. Push your limits, face your fears, test your powers, and discover your abilities. Use adversity like a piece of exercise equipment to make you strong. Discover the truth that was hidden from you: You are stronger than any harm done to you.

Build Self-Esteem. There is no substitute for feeling good about yourself. When you know that you are worthy of love and affection, you will not tolerate mistreatment. Push yourself and grow. Success in the face of challenge communicates powerful messages of competence and worth. Use new experiences to counteract and override old problems. Reach higher, sharpen your skills, increase your abilities. Accept only those limitations you discover through personal effort and experience. Confronting and overcoming problems strengthens you and increases confidence more than any words of encouragement. Progressive challenges build a self-fulfilling expectation of success. Why do you value yourself? Love yourself because you care, exert yourself, do good things, and affirm life. Love others because it is the greatest ride on Earth.

Imagine. Use imagination to help manage your thinking and solve problems. When used to address psychic illness, irony is part of its appeal: some of the same tactics that made you ill can be reversed and used as they were meant—to make you well. The unconscious mind cannot distinguish between fantasy and reality. As far as your unconscious mind is concerned, a well-imagined, successful experience is no different from reality. Mental rehearsals allow you to experiment, improve performance, and try options without risk. Imagine yourself engaging and overcoming difficult situations. Rehearse new tasks, struggles, and triumphs in your mind until they become familiar, everyday things. Choose what instructions you will hear and act upon, drowning out old, irrelevant commands based on habit and fear. Replace negative internal dialogue with positive internal dialogue. Use imagination to explore where you want to go and how you will get there.

Live in the Present. Life is a meditation, and living in the present takes you out of the past. Do one thing at a time and do it well. Practice mindfulness and strive to live each moment to the fullest. Depression dwells in the past; anxiety fantasizes about tomorrow. Life happens today, in the present, and this is where you want to live. The past and future are illusions. Your actions now are the best therapy for your past and the best preparation for your future. Do not live in the past or for tomorrow. They do not exist. Live each day to the fullest, for a good life is nothing more than a series of well-lived days.

Be Open to Change. Being hurt and playing the victim is not the answer. Becoming angry, controlling, compulsive, or addicted is not the answer. Power, money, sex, control, status, revenge: these are not answers. They are substitutes that can never give you what you need. Your answers are more enjoyable than these stupid, stopgap, mind-numbing, soul-killing frauds. Don't change for others. Listen to your instincts. Trust your heart. Believe. Your senses were given to you for a reason. Use them. Learn from them. Change and grow with them. Approach each situation, each person, each day with a fresh mind. Be ready to think and feel things you never thought or felt before. Expect nothing but surprise.

Pursue Goals. Goals point your mind forward and focus on worthy destinations; they structure thinking and behavior in constructive ways. Healing from psychic illness involves more than solving problems. Our world becomes what we focus on, and a problem-oriented mindset is a poor strategy for walking through the world. You don't need to solve all your problems. Embrace the problems you cannot solve and use them to help you grow. Happiness is not the absence of problems. Happiness and unhappiness are manufactured inside our minds, chosen interpretations of events. Living well requires enduring motivation and meaningful goals that challenge us and help us grow. Engage the reward circuits in your brain. Figure out what you want, and go after it with everything you've got.

Be Flexible. If you adapted to toxic environments in the past, the question becomes, when your situation changes and provides new freedom, can you adapt and take advantage of the new opportunities around you? Mental health requires flexible thinking and behavior. Open yourself to new experiences and seek new ways to do things. Build a large repertoire of activities that allow you to do any one thing in many ways. Learn from experience, change your actions, and grow. Avoid emotional investment in being right. Flexibility communicates goodwill and demonstrates you will meet others halfway. Open your mind, heart, and eyes, look for opportunities to grow, and use them.

FIXED MINDSET

- Avoids risks.
- Sees problems as burdens.
- Avoids challenges.
- Gives up easily.
- Sees effort as unpleasant.
- Ignores problems and repeats mistakes.
- Feels threatened by others' success.
- Creates fatalistic thinking and feelings of helplessness.
- Produces underachievement and a plateaued life trajectory.

GROWTH MINDSET

- Accepts risks.
- Sees problems as challenges.
- Embraces challenges.
- Persists.
- Sees effort as a path to mastery.
- Learns from experience and changes actions accordingly.
- Feels inspired by others' success.
- Provides a sense of personal power and agency.
- Produces increasing achievement and an upward life trajectory.

Think Strategically. Mental health is about the strategies we use to meet our needs and solve our problems. Some strategies are effective and healthy; some are not. Before adopting a strategy, try it inside your head and imagine the likely result. After implementing a strategy, evaluate its effectiveness. How did it work? Use your imagination to simulate real-world conditions and determine your best course of action. Many everyday decisions involve mental modeling and strategic thinking. When you ask yourself if an article of clothing would be appropriate in a certain situation, you probably imagine yourself wearing it and other people's responses. Chess also involves strategic thinking, choosing your moves based on your opponent's anticipated response. Before adopting a strategy, imagine the likely result. Strategic thinking costs nothing. It performs experiments without risk, reduces failures, and allows you to quickly change, adapt, and grow, increasing your abilities and freedom.

Practice Skills for Dealing with Difficult People. Difficult people are a fact of life. You have met them before, and you will meet them again. This shouldn't be, but it is not enough to repeatedly act surprised and protest the injustice. We need practical skills for dealing with difficult people. It is beyond the scope of this book to describe these skills here, but a search for the words "difficult people" will yield various media in this growing genre.

Be Honest with Yourself. Meeting one person who admits their mistakes and another who does not, we can assume that the first stands taller than the last, for they have grown with experience. Whatever you do, don't lie to yourself. You have enough problems without that. It is never advantageous to lie to yourself. Honesty is crucial to growth. It allows you to see clearly and act effectively. Examine the choices you've made and the choices before you now. What do you want? What does it require?

Recognize Your Limitations. Our limitations define our abilities, and we cannot know one without the other. A realistic assessment of your abilities expands your capabilities. It makes your actions effective, based upon a correct appraisal of yourself and your situation. Knowing your limitations gives you strength, and the ability to ask for needed help opens vast resources. Keep your ego out of problems, and don't base your self-esteem upon the lies of psychic illness. You don't have to prove anything to anybody. Humility provides detachment and clarity of vision. It disconnects self-esteem from the lies of psychic illness and disengages you from other people's psychopathology. Your actions should fit your environment, so be realistic. Set attainable goals and work within your limits while steadily pushing to expand them. Pick your battles and use your energy wisely. Make every effort count. We don't need to be perfect, and mistakes are a normal and necessary part of growing. When defeated, keep trying. Find your limits, know them well, and push past them.

> A man's reach should exceed his grasp, or what's a heaven for?
> —Robert Browning

Strive. We grow by pushing ourselves, reaching beyond our grasp. Growing is a stretch, and striving is therapeutic. It focuses on unrealized possibilities, expands your limits, and gives hope. By achieving goals that once seemed unattainable, you learn firsthand about your strengths. Strive. Your present abilities are benchmarks to surpass. Push yourself on all fronts: exercise your body, challenge your mind, open your heart, wrestle with moral dilemmas, and reach for things greater than yourself. Growing feels good. Savor it. Enjoy the firming of your body, stimulation of your brain, growth of your heart, and increase of your abilities. We are plastic creatures able to remake ourselves through action. Place yourself in challenging situations, push yourself, and grow.

Laugh. Many comedians have had difficult personal histories that taught them to use humor to cope with adversity. Laughter is medicine that triggers biochemical changes to help defeat pain and depression (Mobbs et al., 2003). When people laugh at their problems, we understand they are stronger than the troubles before them. Laughter moves us. It can transform pain into pleasure and expand your control. Humor diminishes psychic illness by reframing, deflecting, deflating, releasing, and giving perspective to pain. Shared humor connects us to others (Provine, 1996). Laughter reassures us that we are vital beings who can overcome our problems. Humor can free us to love when we feel our worst. Laughing at ourselves and the absurdity of our situation allows us to step outside our problems and momentary cares.

Create. The urge to produce is a primary drive with obvious survival value. Creativity and productivity organize thinking and behavior in pursuit of desired goals, making them naturally therapeutic. Creative acts establish you as a powerful and vital being with mastery of your situation. Create, produce, and grow. Put your energy into music, writing, painting, cooking, pottery, gardening, coding, carpentry, and crafting. Parent, repair, restore, heal, design, nurture, and build. Raise healthy children, help others, and contribute to your community.

Give. When people hit bottom, when life has picked them clean and left them nothing, they often behave oddly. They start giving. They help others. They give their last dime, last morsel of food, a prized possession, their understanding, time, attention, and care. One man, a hitchhiker I picked up, was homeless, filthy, and disheveled, with nothing to his name but a pocket copy of the New Testament, which he attempted to give me after I had done nothing more than share a ride and speak kindly to him. Once, when hitchhiking with a friend, a woman picked us up. She trembled as she explained she never picked up hitchhikers. She was driving to the courthouse to sign divorce papers. She had hit bottom, and here she was, giving a ride to strangers to help us out. A man in poverty inhabiting a tenant trailer in a Florida orange orchard offered me the only food he had, a few unpopped kernels of corn in the bottom of a pan, apologizing as he handed it to me with a slight bow of his head and uplifted eyes. When things like this happen, you are in the presence of something special. Psychologists call this altruism and classify it as a defense, but it is much more. After no small measure of astonishment and admiration, I believe that I understand.

These people inhabit the edge of life and don't want to go over. Their reaching out is an invitation for us to reach back. It is an offer to connect, a mastery of their situation, an affirmation of life. Giving bestows a richness unrelated to material wealth that connects us to others and brings us to life. At some unspoken level, when we hit bottom, we understand that giving completes and heals us. Unselfish giving is an investment that returns even more. Help one another. Lift each other up. We're all we've got. Giving is a form of love that transforms all involved, a simple transaction that reproduces and multiplies goodwill. There are many forms of wealth, not all of which are rooted in this world.

Aspire. Your energies are greater, more focused, and more productive when you have selected a destination and know where you are going. Aspire. Aspirations make a map of your life. They give you direction and guide choices to help you find your way. Healthy aspirations activate and uplift. They boost immunity and help us heal.

Persist. Psychic illness instills feelings of helplessness and hopelessness to sabotage growth and keep us trapped. Persistence helps you escape. If you haven't known defeat, you haven't tried hard enough. The number of times that you have fallen is not important. What is important is how many times you have gotten back up and tried again. You are trapped in dark troubles, your way uncertain. You will try many paths, most of which will lead to no end. Your efforts must be many, for defeats will be frequent. To find your way from these shores, you must push yourself harder and longer than you ever thought possible. You must persist.

Most worthy efforts require many trials, and tenacity sees us through the inevitable disappointments and setbacks that are a part of growing. Success requires that we survive defeat, learn from experience, and try something else. Exploring new ground, your actions are part trial and part error. Do not let the errors of your trials discourage you. When you get stuck, try something else. Nothing guarantees success, but things will not change unless you persist.

Persist. When you fall down, when you are *knocked* down, get up and try again. Take chances. You are strong. Falling while trying hurts less than staying down and giving up. Defeat teaches that you are sturdier than you imagined. Effort makes you stronger, more capable, and provides valuable information about your abilities and the things you struggle against. Unsuccessful attempts are not failures. They are growth steps that bring you closer to solutions. Each unsuccessful effort makes you stronger.

Persist. Transmitters told you that you were helpless and things were hopeless. They lied. These people are afraid of you. They know what you can do. Don't make your efforts hostage to immediate success. It took time to get you into this, and it will take time to get you out. Health is a process, not an event. It requires continued vigilance, looking for opportunities even in problems. Especially in problems. If one thing doesn't work, try something else.

Persist. Fight the good fight, choose your efforts carefully, give them variety, and keep a good heart. Put yourself in encouraging environments and rewarding situations. Use frustration and distress to make you strong. Take satisfaction from each forward step. Do not fear defeat. There are many battles, and none are decisive. The point is not to win but to continue trying. Do this, and you will find your way. Choices feed evil, and resisting evil starves it.

Assess Trustworthiness and Take Appropriate Risks. Psychic illness betrays trust to damage existing relationships and our ability to form new relationships. This makes us isolated, risk-averse, hypervigilant, cautious, and weak. The solution to betrayal is not to become mistrustful but to learn to assess trustworthiness. The lies of psychic illness make this an important life skill. Untrustworthy people use words to trigger emotions and distract you from their behavior. Look at their history and watch for behavior that contradicts speech. Lies are tools for extracting resources. People lie because they want something, and they don't think they'll get it by telling the truth. Lies are told with words but exposed by behavior. Behavior is an X-ray of the soul, revealing internal thoughts, feelings, beliefs, and intent. Talk is cheap, but behavior tells you everything you need to know about a person. Assess trustworthiness, believe behavior, take appropriate risks, and grow.

Find Corrective Experiences. The power of an experience diminishes over time as we encounter new and different experiences. What is learned can be unlearned and replaced with new learning. New experiences can heal old wounds. Sickened by environment, experience, and choice, these things can also heal us. Use good things to crowd out bad things. Use connection to repair disconnection. Find people and create situations that make you feel alive and vital. You need a place that fits you, not arbitrary obstacles to struggle against. Your surroundings should not wear you down or hold you back. You need things that build you up and move you forward, that meet your needs and nurture you, a wholesome environment that affirms your dignity, supports your purpose, and rewards your choice of life. These things heal the problems of the past.

Build Healthy Relationships. Relationships are the source of our greatest joys and worst sorrows. Relationships cause psychic illness, and they can cure it. Healthy relationships undo the effects of a bad past. They rebuild trust, strength, and love. New relationships expose us to different ways of living, allow us to try new activities, and put our past in perspective. They can rework and resolve old problems in new ways. Healthy relationships heal us.

That man is the richest whose pleasures are the cheapest.
—Henry David Thoreau

Simplify. As our material culture has changed, we have changed. During the past century, the role of money and material possessions has evolved from fulfilling basic material needs to providing comfort, luxury, entertainment, distraction, security, status, love, sex, power, acceptance, and belonging. We no longer grunt and pound our chests; we flaunt expensive cars, clothes, and homes. We've made acquisition a competitive sport (Veblen, 1899/1994). We use money now not to meet our needs but to indulge our desires. This is unhealthy. This is no basis for a healthy psyche, functioning society, or sustainable ecosystem.

Where will it end? When will it be enough? We idolize wealth, power, and status and use marketability as the standard by which everything is measured. Idolatry leads us away from ourselves, each other, and God. Our greatest need is for love, but judging by our expenditure of time and energy, love is routinely subordinated to frivolity and ego. Material wealth can only satisfy a few basic human needs. Once these needs are met, additional wealth can eventually begin to interfere with meeting our needs. It is too easy to use wealth as a substitute, taking us from the source of life and shielding us from the consequences of our actions. Money is not the root of all evil, but it should be handled carefully and cautiously. Money can be dangerous. Ownership involves relationship. It is a two-way street. Be careful, or your money and possessions may come to own *you*.

No shopping, house, portfolio, car, or clothes can fill the emptiness inside you. Material possessions cannot meet your greatest needs. Substitutes temporarily anesthetize and then wear off, leaving an even larger money habit and debt hangover, pushing you to repeat the cycle. Money doesn't make you rich, but it can make you poor. Excess possessions—more than you need or can use—take you away from life. Our appetites can betray and control us. They can become weapons, turned and used against us.

Simplify, simplify (Thoreau, 1854). Having few needs brings its own kind of wealth. Discard clutter that gets in the way of living. Cast off what you do not need and will not use. Filter out the extraneous and irrelevant. Make your world knowable and reliable. Live simply, direct, and plain. Taste the unadorned essence of life. Be frugal, but give yourself what you need. Live between deprivation and indulgence, what Aristotle (350 B.C.E., 1926) called the golden mean and Buddha called the middle way, and your appetites will no longer control you. Reduce life to its basic elements. Consciously select the technologies you use to fit your environment. Focus on one thing at a time. Multitasking is not a virtue; it is a flight from awareness.

Prioritize things that connect you to life. Want less and live more. Monitor your desires for strains of compulsion, distraction, and addiction. Get off the buy-borrow treadmill, take control of your personal economy, and stop slaving for advertisers. Consider every purchase not in terms of dollars but in terms of the time you spent to acquire those dollars (Dominguez & Robin, 1992) and costs to the environment (Hawken, 2010) and other people. How much of your life are you willing to trade for pretty things you do not need, that degrade your living environment or require that others toil in unjust circumstances? Live in the present. Greed produces its own kind of poverty, not physical but spiritual and moral. It hollows you out. Acquisitiveness and consumerism are no way to live. They cannot feed your appetite for life. Once you have food in your stomach, clothes on your back, a roof over your head, and a ballot box down the street, material possessions take on different meanings and become like a tapeworm, eating your sustenance from within. There is more to life than acquisition and consumption. Once your physical needs are met, use your time and energy not to acquire but to experience.

Choose Life. If the problem is our separation from life through awareness, then the question must be, how can we reunite with creation? There can be but one answer: We must choose life. Psychic illness may be a disease, but it is mediated by choice. Freedom and choice removed us from nature, and only they can reunite us. In all of creation, only human choice lies beyond God's gate. Choices challenge us every day of our lives, modern temptations with powers to separate us from creation. There is no greater affirmation than for free and aware beings to count themselves with the forces of life.

Choice is the only thing we control, our most powerful activity that determines what we become. Good choices lead us to life. When we choose life, psychic illness loses an important ally and is starved. Life-denying experiences and choices make us ill. Life-promoting experiences and choices heal and strengthen us and help us grow. Life is the source of all Earthly value. All value is derived from life. Psychic illness has no power and must draw its energy from the denial of life. It is a parasite that sucks energy from entities more alive than itself. Shake it off.

Make your actions congruent with the life around you. It is not any one choice we make but a series of choices over time that transforms us and ends evil. The cumulative effect of your actions is that you either deny or affirm life. Your choice is to feed the virus or feed life. The one you feed wins. We stand forever at the crossroads of life and death. These are not things once done and then gone but an unending series of choices culminating in the present moment. Choose life, and you change the world.

Love conquers all things.

—Virgil

These things I command you, that ye love one another.

—John 15:17

Love. Love connects us, heals us, and makes us strong. Love and evil both appreciate and hunger for the life in others but differ in strategies for connection. Evil tries to smother and steal life because it assumes that living is a zero-sum game and theft is the only way that it can get what it needs and wants. Love sees other, more gentle, pleasant, and effective possibilities: caring, creating, sharing, and nurturing. This is cooperation, not control. Love works; evil fails. This truth was hidden from you. Bells are ringing, doors are open, people are gathering. It is time to come home.

Make Your World Larger. We make our world small without knowing it, leaving us the scraps of life, unaware of what life could be. Our spiritual maturity is measured by how wide our arms reach, the extent to which we embrace people different from ourselves. *The Autobiography of Malcolm X* describes his transformation from selfishness and spiritual poverty, gradually expanding his identity until it included all humanity. At some point in our journey, we realize we are part of something far greater than our solitary selves. The healing receiver comes to terms with his hurt, anger, and desire for revenge. He faces these things, weighs them, and lets them go. He recognizes his potential for harm, sees he is not so different from those who hurt him, and uses this knowledge to put his life on a different path. The sequential books of the Bible reflect this evolution of human morality and consciousness: from exclusive to inclusive groups, from condemning to forgiving attitudes, vengeance to compassion, and selfishness to redeeming love. It is humankind growing up.

Psychic illness constructs illusions of alienation, separation, division, and strife to gain power and control. We pursue so-called "personal" interests, deluded that we compete for limited resources. See the illusion of separateness and confront your capacity for harm. How will you connect with other life? Our interests are not exclusive. They are reciprocal, bound up and inseparable. It is never in our interest to exploit or harm others. There is a better way. Malice harms all involved. Blind to the mutuality of our interests, we have hurt too many innocents, fought too many battles, and exploited too many of our own. All wars are civil wars. Man is a family, and we are its brothers, sisters, parents, and children. We have no enemies but our own malice, fear, ignorance, and greed. It is time to redesign our cultures so that our interests combine, not conflict.

Having come to awareness, our task is to expand our circle of caring to include all humanity and all life. Open your eyes: all is connected. The individualism and egocentricity of the past 500 years, having contributed so much to the economic and political advancement of that time, are now archaic. No more of defining ourselves in opposition to one another; we are of one planet. To survive, we must change. We must grow. There is no room for racism in a healthy heart. Connect. Care. See the unity of all people. Expose illusions of separateness and see the forces that devour life for the parasites they are. We are on this world to overcome the superficial differences painted before us, to love one another, and regain the connection with other life lost through our ascent to consciousness. There are many ways up the mountain (Kornfield, 1993), and whether we call this al-Islam, Brahman, nirvana, salvation, or Yahweh, our work on this world is to complete the circle back and make us whole with life once more. Our fates have always been bound together, but we forgot this when we rose to consciousness. Well, no more.

There was a time when the world's cultures had much less contact, and we could afford to act as separate entities. That time has passed. Our cultures, economies, and nations connect more each day. Soon they will weave one fabric stretched across the globe. Our borders become less relevant with the passing of each month, and the thought of any nation acting without regard for others becomes less rational each year. Once, the world was made of countless cultures, economies, and political entities. Soon it will contain one system, a confederation of people woven together, interacting and connecting to form a larger organism. We are one species. It is time we act like it. We shall live together or die together. Whichever we choose, we will do it together. There are no other paths before us.

Practice Stewardship. We are caretakers, charged with protecting and nurturing life until passing it on to the next generation. Our choices affect not just ourselves; they affect those who follow. We have responsibilities. Stewards of this planet and our cultures, we inhabit a brief moment in the river of life as it flows through space and time to new generations and new places. Our institutions require watchful tending and care to remain healthy. They guide and protect us. We must guide and protect them.

Cultivate Wonder and Awe. You see it in young children. They begin life with wide eyes and bright smiles, beaming with life. But time passes, they see some things, learn some things, they grow into adults, and when you look at some faces, the light is gone, the fire out, the ashes cold. Their woeful countenance betrays a weariness heavier than any millstone. How can this be?

To be aware of life's magic is to appreciate its unrealized potential. Wonder and awe increase our perception and understanding. They open us to new experiences and possibilities. Who is more expert in wonder and awe than a child? Children are wise because they have no preconceived notions about the world. They are wise not in the ways of the world but in the ways of life. So young, they are that much closer to the source of life. Naturally honest and valuing life, we can learn from them.

Open your eyes to the everyday miracles around you. Cultivate wonder and awe. Focus on the positive, give thanks, and revere life's mysteries. There is magic in this world if we open ourselves to it. Recall the time before you were prejudiced by worldly knowledge and see once more through young eyes. Stop making assumptions. Return to the wisdom of simple, unadulterated experience, alive to each moment. Go out and play. Open your heart to the life around you and live with the wonder of a child.

Be Kind. We never know the end of even our most minor actions. Given the right time and place, a smile, a word of encouragement, or a simple acknowledgment of one's humanity can turn a disastrous chain of events into an affirmation of life. We feed each other, and there are no small acts of kindness. They are noticed. They make a difference. Practice random acts of kindness, and when someone does you a kindness, pay it forward. Evil is infectious; goodness is too. We don't need to be perfect. The rule is simple: give better than you got, and you change the world. When we all do this, evil will die a natural death, and the world will pass into a higher order of being.

Others look to you now for their protection and guidance. Do not make your pain their pain. Teach your children to value life. Get involved. Show that you care and make a difference. We belong to each other. We are responsible for each other. We are here to lift each other up. Refuse to tolerate exploitation and harm. Protect vulnerable people. Your pain is healed by restoring the world to its natural order and making things right for future generations. You are breeding life. Your hands and your heart can change the world.

Give Better than You Got. Your ancestors were alive one thousand, ten thousand, one hundred thousand years ago. They learned some things. They chose some things. They taught some things. Some of this has come to you now. What will you choose? What will you teach? Fight harm with comfort and hurt with love. Love is the ultimate medicine, more powerful than the most potent antibiotic. In loving we are saved, freed from the bonds of our solitary existence, and connected to life once more. Solve your problems as they were meant: reach, connect, care. Put the energy from your pain into healthy, life-promoting action. This is the secret that was hidden from you: we solve these problems with love.

Follow Your Dreams. Your dreams are your innermost sense of possibility, truer than any circumstances forced upon you. They reveal your potential and light your path to higher ground. Listen to your dreams. You dream for a reason. Dreams give hope and energy. They lift us out of our circumstances and focus activity on future goals. Follow your dreams and work to make them a reality.

Choose Well

The most important issue facing us today is how we define what it is to live well. How we answer this question radically affects every aspect of our lives. It determines our standard of living, our health, prosperity, the quality of our environment, our freedom, and future. Will we live free through rational choice and love, or be ruled by manipulation, fear, and impoverishment? Our numbers now are so great and technologies so powerful, that how we answer this question will determine the fate of life on Earth.

Many of today's challenges are problems of lifestyle. We are confused, defining happiness as money, power, status, consumption, and control. We slave at jobs, bicker and fight, destroy our health, and degrade our environment—all in the pursuit of happiness. But we are not happy. We are addicted, impoverished, and afraid. The more we chase after what we have been told is the good life, the more happiness eludes us. Our emotions, relationships, health, standard of living, and the Earth suffer as a result. Our economies are increasingly indebted and unsustainable. Workers and resources are becoming scarce, the environment is stressed, the economy is shaky, debts are high, and savings are low. Necessities are increasingly unaffordable, products and work are less safe, wages haven't budged for decades, and political discourse is increasingly aggressive and disconnected from reality. Our quality of life is deteriorating. This is not the life we were promised.

We've been lied to, told that freedom and happiness come from vice, wealth, power, status, and control. That lie enslaves us. It has enriched and empowered generations of sociopaths who care nothing for our well-being or our planet's health. That lie jeopardizes the very things it promises. We are promised freedom and good lives by corrupted people who rob us of our freedom and destroy our quality of life (2 Peter 2:19). There is a better way.

You can adopt a lifestyle that helps free you from being controlled by others and many of society's problems, even as you remain actively engaged, a path of better living that simultaneously transforms yourself and the world. Live simply. Free yourself from excessive possessions, dysfunctional relationships, needless constraints, exploitative economies, and unhealthy cultural influences. Stop serving the virus. Affirm life by finding and exercising your power. Shake off socially encouraged passivity and assumptions about what you require to live well. Prosper by following a rational path of freedom and awareness. Disengage from psychic illness and engage instead with the best that life has to offer. Adopt a healthy mindset and healthy behavior.

Value facts over ideology and go where the truth takes you. Be flexible in your thinking and behavior. Consciously choose how you think and what you do. Experiment. Try new thoughts and behaviors and evaluate the results. What works? What doesn't? Learn from experience and grow. Identify your assumptions and discard those that prove untrue. See the two paths of existence, having and being (Fromm, 1976). The first is possessive and acquisitive. It leads to controlling and controlled relationships that take us away from life. It makes you weak, vulnerable, and hungry. The second is experiential. It fosters connection and growth. It makes you strong, resilient, and fulfilled.

Believe that a better world is possible, and work toward it. Value growth—positive change that benefits you and others. Growth is always possible. Value life more than objects. Possessions are means to ends, not ends in themselves. They become addictive. Have and use possessions, but do not make them the focus of your life. Experience—what you perceive, think, feel, and do—is the essence of life. A good life is filled with good experiences. This is the better way. Wealth and possessions can contribute to positive experiences only to the extent that they meet your basic needs. Beyond that, they can poison you and interfere with your ability to experience pleasure and live well. Beware of shiny things.

My living well does not require your loss. That would be parasitism. In healthy relationships, what benefits one benefits others, knitting us together, strengthening each of us, and improving conditions for all. The path of living well is simple: be kind, compassionate, responsible, and courageous. Live simply and directly. Apply yourself. Strive, reach, and struggle. Use moderate stress to challenge yourself, stimulate growth, and make yourself free. Growth has no end, and it feels great.

We have everything we need to make this planet a paradise. No poverty, hunger, or war. Health. Education. Safety. Sanitation. Clean water. Affordable housing and energy. Reliable income and good food. Community. Prosperity and quality of life for all. We lack only the will. Rationally change your thinking and behavior. This ability is within you, has always been within you, even when dormant. Awaken it. Shake off your chains and transform this world.

Do not listen to people who conspire to make you poor. Have a mindset of abundance and gratitude, not poverty and hunger. Work with what you have. Focus more on pursuing positives and less on avoiding negatives. Let good crowd out the bad. Be politically active. Educate yourself on issues, vote, run for office, and hold your representatives accountable. Get signatures and put initiatives on the ballot. On all levels, do what you can to make the world a better place. Stand up for others. Discuss issues and educate yourself to better understand the world and all that happens around you. Enjoy growth and seek a better way. Strive for a positive cash flow, earning more than you spend. This frees you from the tyranny of debt and uncertainty. Live the good life one

> **HOW TO HEAL PSYCHIC ILLNESS**
>
> 1. Become aware of the past in the present.
> 2. Believe that change is possible.
> 3. Choose to change.
> 4. Make your pain work for positive, needed change that affirms life.
> 5. Disengage from Psychic illness. Do not let others hurt you, do not hurt others, do not tolerate the hurting of others.
> 6. Respond to your preferences and meet your needs.
> 7. Deal with real problems, not substitutes.
> 8. Choose healthy values that affirm life.
> 9. Surround yourself with healthy people.
> 10. Let go of the past.
> 11. Give better than you got.
> 12. Follow your dreams.

experience at a time. Live well in the present, and the future tends to take care of itself.

Work to create a just world. When you look at others, see more similarities than differences and seek common ground. Build bridges and alliances—these make you strong and wealthy in all the ways a person can be wealthy. Our living environment feeds us. Savor experience, be honest, and face hard truths.

Do not avoid problems; pitch in and work on them. Pain and distress signal the existence of problems and the need for change. Problems are opportunities to grow. Fight for what you believe in. Do not tolerate injustice or exploitation. Use moderate, normal challenges to make you strong. Enjoy them and the growth they bring. Strive to do better. Wrestling with problems makes us grow, and growth feels wonderful. Learn to entertain yourself and enjoy most situations you encounter. Engage life with your hands, head, and heart. Money is a means, not an end. Shun debt when possible, recognizing it as a form of servitude.

Lifestyle is powerful medicine for preventing and treating many chronic diseases and improving your quality of life. Make diet, rest, and exercise the foundation of your health. Consciously bring good things into your life and the lives of others. Vote with your money and use this to reward right action. Fight for what is just and strive to make the world more livable. This is noble work. Universal safety, education, and healthcare benefit us all. These are investments in people, our most valuable resource. All change begins within. Change yourself, and you change how others respond to you. Change how others respond to you, and you change the world.

This is an ancient message from Abraham, Buddha, Jesus, Muhammad, and countless others. We walk in the footsteps of giants. This message resonates now because of the time we live in. Follow this path and thrive. Help others, care for others, and prosper. Your actions ripple out and back to you in a thousand ways. This is the path before you, the life you are meant to live. Begin your change by fitting parts of this into your life and watch what happens. Examine the results. If you find value, try some more. Feed the living world around you. There are two paths, two strategies. Choose well.

Chapter 4

PREVENTION

In the ways of Nature, there is no evil to be found.
—Marcus Aurelius

Preventives of evil are far better than remedies; cheaper and easier of application, and surer in result.
—Tryon Edwards

This chapter summarizes some of the systemic institutionalized problems now driving psychic illness and cultural strategies that suppress it. These are discussed in greater depth in Chapter Eight, *Prevention*, found in *Psychic Illness: The Rise and Fall of Evil on Earth* (Sweitzer, 2001 & manuscript in preparation).

> **PSYCHIC ILLNESS IS VULNERABLE**
>
> - Must hide in darkness and deception.
> - Thrives on fear and superstition; fades under dispassionate examination.
> - A viral Parasite, it has no powers of its own.
> - Infectious diseases are relatively easy to control.

We are told that it is human nature to exploit and harm. It is a seductive argument. "My behavior is normal and therefore excusable. What do you expect? I'm only human." The virus normalizes mistreatment and tells us it is inevitable. "You cannot help yourself. This is who you are. There is no escape, no alternative, so don't even try." Beware of those who tell you to abandon hope, for Hell is sure to follow (Alighieri, 1320/2013).

We are, by nature, neither good nor evil. We are what we choose to be, and the world is what we make it. We are free. Culture and psyche are software, and we are programmable. There is no innate human nature. Evil is not baked into our souls. It is a parasite latched onto us that can be starved and shed. We can become our own worst nightmare, or we can make a paradise of Earth and live amazing lives. The choice is ours.

Psychic illness is found only in humans and is unknown to nature. All other species manage to live without it. It is not a necessary part of life. What we call evil could not have existed before we invented culture. If we date the beginning of human culture as the first physical evidence of our use of tools, then evil is less than three million years old, less than 1/1,000th of Earth's existence. Evil is a recent phenomenon on Earth, a young organism confined to a single species, and it requires highly specific and unnatural conditions to live. Many people manage to live mostly without it, and it varies greatly by time and place, revealing the enormous role of environmental factors and its susceptibility to alteration of these variables. Psychic illness is vulnerable to the tools of science and may even be eradicated. Remember smallpox?

There is nothing to suggest, no reason to believe, that evil is a necessary part of human being. What is made can be unmade. Men and women created evil, and men and women can dismantle it. Evil is not some intrinsic part of the human condition. It is not natural or necessary. It is an external parasite, an alien. We are not born with it. It is acquired. This doesn't have to be. We don't have to feed it. We don't have to live with it. We don't have to die with it. There was a time not so long ago when evil did not walk this Earth, and as fantastic as it sounds, that time may come again.

The Book of Genesis describes the behavioral transmission of evil: it passed from the serpent to Eve, from Eve to Adam, to Cain and Abel and all their descendants. Both Christianity and the theory of behavioral virology see evil as transmitted through behavior. Evil is not fate; it is choice. When we are no longer exposed to evil, when we stop choosing evil, when we stop feeding evil, evil becomes extinct. There is a path to the end of this.

Let's try a thought experiment. Imagine a child born into a situation where she is wanted and loved. The adults in her life are not perfect, but more often than not, they model functional and loving relationships. Her basic needs are reasonably met, and the only hardships she might repeatedly encounter are occasional accidents and illness, life's normal difficulties, and reasonable and healthy challenges she and her parents choose to advance her life or help others. She is not regularly exposed to pathological behavior. She is not repeatedly thrust into dilemmas of artificial, made-up problems. No one is plotting to take her down. She is not spoiled and has no consistent incentives to act badly. There are many incentives to act rationally, respectfully, fairly, playfully, creatively, with humor and love. Her reasonable goals are often attainable. This goes on for generations, and her descendants are surrounded by others who encounter similar conditions. What happens to evil then, when there is nothing left for it to feed on?

Evil is a dysfunctional problem-solving strategy, a response to contrived, man-made situations and problems. What happens when these no longer exist? We end evil by starving it and removing the corrupt incentives for it we've installed in our culture. We quit evil by denying it habitat and refusing to feed, model, or transmit it. We displace evil by providing more effective and pleasant ways of addressing life's challenges. We move beyond evil by providing alternatives that render it unnecessary and obsolete. We lose our need of it. We outgrow it. Certainly, this is a phenomenal undertaking. But the fact that we can imagine it raises the possibility that it can be done. We imagined many things in the past that seemed fantastic, preposterous, utterly impossible to accomplish. And then we did them. Why not this? We are immensely powerful, far more than this parasite virus. We have enormous problems that require equally enormous solutions. This is a time to think big. Another world is possible. If we hold to this vision, it will put us on a better path.

Promote Responsibility and Accountability

Free people live healthy lives because they choose to do so, because it is in their interest and the most attractive alternative available to them. A free society is made of socialized individuals who choose to act responsibly, not subjects who forcibly submit to codified laws. Healthy societies work not because their people fear breaking laws but because they choose to act in ways that benefit both themselves and the commonweal. Their citizens are more free than a society that bans books but permits advertising in schools and ends up with incarcerated criminals unable to function without external limits coercing their behavior. Informal social influence is more effective than legal sanction and often renders legal interventions unnecessary. People remain free and are more likely to act in a desirable manner of their own volition. They have dignity, and they have choice. Legal sanction should not be our first defense against undesirable activity. Infectious misbehavior begs for prevention.

Human rights are inalienable, but they mean nothing when individuals and cultures ignore them. Responsibility is social glue that holds a society together, a social compact based on reciprocity. There can be no rights without responsibility; the two are inseparable. Responsibility enforces rights. Your rights are my responsibility, and my rights are your responsibility. You and I stand back-to-back, guarding each other's interests. If you respect me and I respect you, we both enjoy rights created by each other's behavior. Responsibility requires that we guard other people's rights as fiercely as our own. If we do not protect other people's rights, how can we expect them to protect ours? If we fail to do this, no one has rights, and none are free. It is unavoidable that other people's rights limit our rights.

There are limits to freedom. When your actions are unhealthy, your chances of survival are reduced. It's a fact of nature. If your actions violate other people's rights, you are not exercising freedom; you are taking liberties. Violating other's rights reduces your rights. We live together. If you seek maximum freedom, respecting other people's rights is advantageous to you. It expands your freedom. Human being is about sharing. Healthy cultures protect those who cannot protect themselves. We are a community. We are responsible for each other. We belong to each other. The idea that the psychological health of one person depends to some extent upon the health of others is not some moral platitude; it is an epidemiological fact.

In a democracy, personal responsibility and individual accountability are the foundation of freedom and the guarantors of our liberties. Democracy only works when people are accountable for their actions. When people are irresponsible and unaccountable, they function as parasites, leeching resources from those who are. Democracy is a balancing act of competing interests. The issue is, by what criteria should we balance individual liberty and public interest? It has been said that one person's right to swing her fist ends at the tip of another person's nose. Unrestrained freedom cannot exist within a functioning system, for at some point, one person's unrestrained acts interfere with another person's rights. It is not realistic to value freedom and nothing else. Unrestrained activity is not freedom; it is anarchy and corruption. No one is free in a society of irresponsible and unaccountable people. Responsible individuals are the foundation of a free society. There can be no freedom without responsibility. Responsibility is the foundation of freedom, and individuals who are not accountable jeopardize others' freedom. Irresponsibility destroys democracy. Freedom is purchased with responsibility and accountability; liberty is earned with exertion, struggling against those who would control us.

If we are to limit our freedoms, and we must, is it not best to base those limitations upon consciously chosen rational criteria that support the objectives of our society? Freedom requires that we protect other people's rights as much as our own, that we live by and teach life-promoting values. We can model, encourage, and incentivize healthy beliefs and actions. We can promote responsibility and accountability.

Foster Life-Promoting Values

Life needs more than information to operate. It needs instruction, values that guide us and help us survive. We are moral creatures who live and die by the values we choose. Our values, our choice of life when free and aware, make us human. Values are the lifeblood of a free society, and societies that do not value life cannot last. Cultures that do not value life are doomed by their own want of purpose, direction, and resolve. To survive and live well, we need institutions that value life and environments that reward life-affirming choices. Healthy values and morals are codes of conduct able to resist pathology. They are psychic instructions evolved over time that tell us to align our actions with life. They are cultural antibodies.

All life requires guidance. In the past, we were guided by random mutation, natural selection, and the demands of our environment. Culture introduced values, mores, laws, and institutional incentives to guide us. Laws are institutionalized values, instructions that codify our expectations for each other. But laws should only be used after all other means have failed. Promoting cultural values, norms, and incentives is more reasonable and effective than attempting to legislate morality. Using laws to manage human behavior indicates the failure of other, less coercive means of social guidance. We need healthy, life-promoting values to guide us. So, how do we determine what values are healthy?

The Laws of Life: Using Nature to Determine Healthy Values

> The essence of goodness is preserve life, promote life, help life to achieve its highest destiny. The essence of evil is destroy life, harm life, hamper the development of life.
> —Albert Schweitzer

Nature is not neutral. Nature is highly judgmental and mercilessly destroys organisms that do not live according to its laws. Nature values survival, things that last. Nature values life. Life uses two basic strategies for survival: competition and cooperation.

Every organism uses both to varying degrees. Those who say that altruism, an extended form of cooperation, is ultimately selfish are correct, but they miss the point. Cooperation is reciprocity, an interaction that knits actors together over time. You plow my field, I share my beans. We both gain; it's a better deal. Cooperation connects us to form a larger whole that is stronger, more resilient, and more likely to last than individuals on their own. Nature relentlessly promotes survival, and good things come from it. Computer models that compare the effectiveness of various survival strategies have found that goodness—squishy things like kindness, caring, cooperation, and altruism—enhances survival (Axelrod, 1981). It is an empirically valid strategy for improving one's lot in life. It is to be preserved. Habitual selfishness is not only morally wrong; it is an inferior life strategy that yields inferior results.

Every purposeful act reflects priorities and values. Information and instruction go hand in hand. They are inseparable, the line between them hopelessly blurred. Obviously, there are healthy and unhealthy values. So how do we determine what values are healthy? How do we find our path? Healthy values, expressed as priorities and strategies, guide and protect us. They increase survival. They make us strong and support life. Nature provides countless examples of values and strategies that make organisms healthy and more likely to last. Nature also provides an abundance of cautionary tales of other values and strategies that lead down the short path.

The health of a value is gauged by a simple metric: does it improve our functioning and make us more likely to last? Nature is an efficient, if not ruthless reaper that cares for little else. As it turns out, survival value is as good a measure as you will find to weigh the difference between good and evil. Of course, health and survival are closely related, if not the same. Observations of nature, Earth's foremost expert on survivability, prove informative. Let us now examine what nature teaches us about the strategies and priorities—the values—that promote health and survival.

Survival requires a system. Everything that exists is part of a system composed of interactive parts. Everything is made of several somethings. Biological systems destabilize when they lose parts: the fewer members of a species, the greater the risk of extinction. The fewer species in an ecosystem, the more unstable and imperiled it becomes. In nature, there is strength in numbers, and loners are goners. Nature values interactive, dynamic systems because they increase survivability. Groups are the way to go.

Nations with allies thrive, nations without allies wither.
—James Mattis, former U.S. Secretary of Defense (2022.)

Connections, attachments, and bonds increase strength, health, and survivability. The connection imperative is older than matter (Sweitzer, 2001 & manuscript in preparation) and operates tirelessly even in advanced systems such as psyche and culture. Connections, attachments, and bonds create systems, and systems increase survivability. Intermarriage between groups has long been used to decrease the potential for war. It also increases genetic diversity, which increases survivability. Humans are highly social creatures who form strong emotional and social attachments. We invest our most treasured resources in relationships and enjoy innumerable benefits from cooperative living. Mammals, especially, invest massive resources in relationships. Nature does not invest resources on this scale without a commensurate return. These bonds create strong couples, families, and cultures. Nature values connection because relationships form resilient systems that make us strong, healthy, and more likely to last.

Heterogeneous diversity, as opposed to homogeneous uniformity, increases health and survival. If you have siblings, you are probably quite different from each other, and your parents will tell you that you were born this way. This is nature's plan. On the micro level, sibling variance makes it more likely that at least one child will survive and pass on its parents' genes. On the macro level, populations with greater genetic diversity also fare better. Life promotes diversity. Diversity is beneficial and should be recognized as such in our culture.

When members of a species are not diverse, when they are genetically similar, e.g., through inbreeding, the resulting lack of genetic variation decreases their ability to adapt and survive. Variation within a population increases health and survivability. Monocultures are prone to genetic defects, disease, pests, environmental deterioration, and vicious cycles, making them unhealthy and less likely to last. Intermarriage between groups brings new blood, invigorates a population, and has long been used to combine resources and decrease war. Genetic and cultural diversity increase health and survivability. Diverse ecosystems and populations are more adaptable, resilient, and likely to survive. Cultures that are inclusive, accepting, tolerant, and respectful are more likely to last than cultures that are exclusive, intolerant, rejecting, and disrespectful. Diversity is more than the spice of life; it is an essential ingredient. Nature values and uses diversity because diversity increases health and survival.

Combining strategies of both competition and cooperation maximizes adaptability, health, and long-term survivability. Sometimes, competition is more advantageous; sometimes, cooperation is more advantageous. Often, a combination of the two is most advantageous. The winners in nature's lottery are organisms and cultures that effectively blend these strategies and employ an unbiased, practical preference for whatever works best as conditions change. Strategies that habitually favor competition or cooperation produce suboptimal results, including poor health and decreased chances for survival. Nature plays no favorites. It values and uses both competition and cooperation—blended solutions—as appropriate to the situation because this maximizes health and survivability.

Health and Survival require the use of feedback to coordinate and align actions with environment. We animals possess an entire battery of sensory organs and dedicated brain regions that provide real-time information about our environment and the effectiveness of our actions. Feedback is corrective. It allows us to accommodate and adapt by means other than natural selection. For healthy organisms, there is no blaming or shirking, just ongoing monitoring of one's performance in search of better ways to operate internal processes and respond to one's environment.

Cultures and psyches also require accurate feedback to operate effectively; their actions must be subjected to an ongoing process of conscientious and unbiased self-monitoring, assessment, and review. Cultures and psyches use environmental feedback for situational awareness, defense, mating, feeding, navigation, communication, organization, self-assessment, maintenance, optimal performance, and improvement. None of these are possible without feedback. Feedback informs us of the correctness of our actions—if we are hitting or missing the mark.

Imagine trying to drive a car with its windows, gauges, and warning lights painted over. You are not going anywhere. Imagine trying to learn archery but never looking to see where your arrow landed. You will not improve. Things are not going to change. We need feedback to navigate and survive. Listen to what the world is telling you and learn from experience. Ask, "What am I doing? How is it working?" Organisms that don't use feedback do not last. Failure to properly use feedback is a significant factor in psychic illness. Using feedback to coordinate and align your actions with your environment is essential to health and survival.

Flexibility of function—an unbiased readiness to change oneself or one's environment as needed—promotes health and survival. Humans are masters of both environmental change (manipulating our environment) and personal change (adaptation) to meet our needs and address life's challenges. People can develop an unhealthy bias for environmental or personal change and become inflexible in their choices. Manipulative people can be quite charming and adept at controlling others, while codependent people may be prone to adapt when they encounter problems. Psychopathology often involves a bias toward environmental change or personal change. This results in an overuse of externalizing strategies (e.g., blame, denial, projection, anger, and control) or internalizing strategies (e.g., shame, inappropriate acceptance of responsibility, introjection, anxiety, and passivity.) Some people habitually impose their will on others, whereas others may habitually adapt to other people's demands. The most successful organisms and psyches are flexible and unbiased in their selection of strategies. They are not interested in blaming others or themselves. They want to solve problems, whatever their source. They alter themselves or their environment depending upon the location of the problem. Nature values and flexibly uses both environmental change and adaptation to increase health and survivability.

Cooperative reciprocal relationships maximize the health and long-term survivability of all life's systems and subsystems, including matter, organisms, and species. Nature's systems are composed of co-equal actors participating in cooperative reciprocal relationships. Co-equal atoms combine to form elements. Co-equal molecules combine to form compounds. Cells with only subtle genetic variations, just enough to provide the ability to change over time, form organisms. Atoms, molecules, cells, and elephants are co-equal. Cooperation is used to promote survival as well. Farmers plant seeds, fertilize the soil, and tend crops. In return, they reap food. You feed and house bacteria in your gut; they help you digest your meal and provide you with nutrients, many you can't make for yourself. Plants oxygenate your blood; you feed them carbon dioxide. Over time, actors involved in reciprocal relationships adapt to each other, and the relationships become increasingly beneficial for both. The actors connect and eventually figure out how to work things to their mutual advantage. The relationship becomes cooperative because cooperation helps both survive. Cooperation has survival value.

In cultures and psyches, inequality and strife are parasitic, unhealthy, unnatural, unsustainable, and eventually fatal. They temporarily feed a few at great cost to all. Non-reciprocal strategies that lie, cheat, divide, control, oppress, exploit, and abuse one's counterparts contribute to the downfall of nations and individuals. When societies create monopolies, plutocrats, kleptocrats, tycoons, dictators, and oligarchs, they fail. Inequality is unhealthy for a culture and destroys societies. It devours populations with unnatural disasters of war, famine, and pestilence. Such societies cannibalize themselves. Institutionalized exploitation and abuse are the shadow side of civilization, driven by greed and craving for power and control. They are driven by the virus.

Countries that condone abuse and torture, launch offensive wars, abstain from treaties and international law, and channel disproportionate power and resources to a limited few are unhealthy and unbalanced, destined for systemic failure. Nature teaches us that such systems do not last and are doomed by their isolation, instability, and unresponsiveness to corrective feedback. They are morally wrong and ultimately fail. Such relationships are generally not seen within a species and are evidence of parasite infection: you don't feed on your own kind. That would be suicidal. Exploitation is essentially a mining operation, and all mines eventually fail.

Nature values and uses cooperative reciprocal relationships because they provide survivability for matter, organisms, and species. These relationships provide optimum health and quality of life, and they can go on forever.

> Power tends to corrupt, and absolute power corrupts absolutely.
> —Lord Acton

Nature uses decentralized, distributed decision-making to maximize system health and survivability. All naturally occurring systems begin as disconnected, unrelated parts. The actions of individual actors generate feedback, establishing relationships between actors that eventually connect them. Actors become interactors, forming feedback loops, dependencies, and bonds. Over time, there emerges a larger system containing new and often unforeseeable characteristics, a system that transcends the individual parts that comprise it. Individual agents, operating under simple rules, as a group can generate behavior far beyond their capacity as individuals, and the system's behavior can be far more complex than the behavior of the parts that comprise it (Wolfram, 2002).

A species' need to fit stabilizes an ecosystem. Innumerable actors accommodating each other over time combine to create larger, stable, self-righting systems. Stability comes from the interlocking parts of a system, each with a part to play, each checking the other, each motivated by its own need to fit and survive. Interactions provide feedback, and feedback provides regulation. Through their interactions, parts form connections that eventually balance and stabilize relationships. Combined, they give the Earth equilibrium, homeostasis on a planetary scale.

However, introducing too many, too random, too rapid, and unforeseeable changes destroys parts and destabilizes systems. Random elimination of life's parts (species and individuals) removes the checks they perform (regulation), making ecosystems vulnerable to external influence. Simple, less complex systems are more generalized and tolerant of radical and unpredictable change. When stressed beyond its ability to compensate, life loses parts/species until it again fits its environment. Simplification then stops, and life begins rebuilding diversity and complexity congruent with its new environment. Life has been down this road many times before during numerous extinctions.

During the 1960s, researchers at the Rand Corporation realized that during a nuclear war, the loss of a center of communications would be fatal to a centralized computer network. Their solution was to design a system with no central authority, a peer-to-peer network that would function even with the loss of most of its members. Survivability required that decision-making and control be delegated to co-equal nodes. All would share the same status, each possessing equal authority to create, receive, and pass messages. Survivability required a system with no center and co-equal, interconnected parts. This was the birth of the internet, a robust system designed to survive cataclysmic change and function even after most of its parts were destroyed. It mimics life to survive.

Local, distributed decision-making systems, such as the internet and biological populations, can function even after losing most of their parts. Compared to centralized systems with unequal actors and concentrated cores of decision-making, they make better decisions and are more responsive to change. Schemes that centralize decision-making and control are unnatural and unhealthy. Decapitation, a warfare tactic that destroys an adversary's command and control structures, exploits this vulnerability. Nature does not use centralized command structures because they are vulnerable to decapitation, slow to respond to change, make inferior decisions, poorly coordinate the actions of their many parts, and sub-optimally distribute resources. Instead, nature uses decentralized command structures—colonies of ants, schools of fish, flocks of birds, herds of reindeer—composed of co-equal actors that yield swarm intelligence and make populations and species resilient. Distributing decision-making across many actors makes systems healthy and more likely to last.

Craving for power is a symptom of psychic illness, and systems that concentrate power inevitably become filled by infected people who yearn for it and crave even more (Klaas, 2022). This is poor cultural design. Power comes at other people's expense: people who crave power subordinate other people's interests to their own. We can do better. People who greatly desire power should not hold high office or be trusted with power over others. A pathological desire for power—as exhibited by a person's past behavior, what they have been willing to do to acquire power, or a history of mistreating people or abusing power—should disqualify people from holding positions entrusted with power over others. The risks are too great. Such people crave power to abuse it and parasitize public resources for personal gain. It is time to recognize this form of embezzlement and put an end to such practices.

Examining the political and personal histories of many world leaders, there was ample evidence of their being unfit prior to achieving high office. Had this information been properly responded to, it would have prevented much pain and misery, and history would have been improved. Evil leaves a trail behind it that can be detected, and this can be used to prevent these mistakes of history.

Power and wealth also exert a corrupting influence on individuals, groups, and countries, creating yet another reason they should not be greatly concentrated but dispersed throughout a population. Cultures that greatly concentrate power and wealth are unnatural, unhealthy, and less likely to last. China, Russia, North Korea, and Iran are now experiencing a multitude of self-inflicted wounds and appear disposed to address them through war. Violence is a BBV force multiplier, and most violence and wars are virus-driven.

These countries were brought to this state by unnatural concentrations of power combined with insufficient checks and balances and the inevitable mismanagement that follows. Their way out of this mess is to equitably distribute power and wealth—to implement democratic reforms and social and economic justice. Democratic societies are stronger, more stable, innovative, prosperous, less warlike, and more likely to survive than undemocratic societies. When capitalism works, it does so because it delegates economic decisions to many people. Nature uses cooperative, decentralized, distributed decision-making and control to maximize system health and survivability. This is what works. This is the superior strategy for lasting. This is how we survive.

Slavishly carrying every fertilized egg to term is unnatural and unhealthy, and it decreases the survivability of species. Reproduction is one of the riskiest activities that animals undertake, and nature routinely uses this process as an opportunity to cull the weak and select the strong before significant resources are expended upon unviable offspring and inadequate environments. Nature routinely eliminates organisms in utero that are not developing normally and face poor prospects. This process is normal, natural, and the most frequent cause of human miscarriages. It is responsible for the spontaneous abortion of 40-60% of human fertilized eggs, often before the woman even realizes she is pregnant (Jarvis, 2016). Nature also ends pregnancies when it detects an unfavorable environment for offspring. When a bear becomes pregnant, her fertilized eggs do not immediately develop. Instead, they enter a state of delayed implantation—embryonic diapause—where they remain viable but stop developing. It is not until she begins her winter sleep and has found sufficient resources in her environment to support the offspring that the egg will implant on the uterine wall and begin to grow. When she's found insufficient food in her environment, she absorbs the egg and terminates the pregnancy. Other animals delay or forgo implantation when lactating, as this also signals insufficient resources for pregnancy.

Embryonic diapause is used by about 100 mammal species for health and survival, increasing the odds that offspring will be born into environments that can support them. In humans, malnutrition and low levels of body fat—reliable indicators of environmental insufficiency—trigger miscarriages. Abortion is natural. Abortion is necessary. Natural human abortion occurs nearly as often as human birth. Nature routinely uses abortion to prevent human birth defects and avoid offspring being born into conditions that cannot support them. Slavishly carrying every fertilized egg to term is unnatural and unhealthy; it promotes birth defects and decreases the health and survivability of our species. At a time when we are greatly exceeding the carrying capacity of the planet, forcing people to have children they do not want or cannot carry or care for is irrational and antithetical to life.

Circular material economies are natural and sustainable and promote survivability. We are the only species that creates garbage: the things we touch seem to leave the cycle of life for a very long time. So-called "forever chemicals" or per- and polyfluoroalkyl substances (PFAS) (EPA, 2022), PCBs, certain pesticides, and plastics that now infuse the seas and our tissues are not easily broken down by natural processes and linger in our environment for unnaturally long periods where they do damage. In contrast, nature lets nothing go to waste. Everything is recyclable. Where there is something to be eaten, there is something to eat it. We need to transition from a linear material economy to a circular material economy where design, manufacture, and recycling follow intelligent and funded plans (e.g., deposits included in the purchase price) for each item's constituent parts after its useful life has expired. We also need to tax noxious by-products. This approach becomes increasingly necessary as we poison our environment and our resources dwindle. It reduces environmental toxins and synthetic objects that torment sea creatures. Reducing the variety of materials we produce will allow them to be genuinely recycled, not just melted and mixed.

Instituting an intelligently designed circular economy for manufactured objects will make us and our environment more healthy and more likely to last. Circular is practical and sustainable. Linear is not.

Our continued existence requires that we choose values that support life. There is no other path to survival.

Increase Public Awareness of Psychic Illness

It has been recognized throughout history that managing consciousness is essential to happiness. Ideas compete in a Darwinian process, driving the evolution of thought and culture. The requirements for managing consciousness change as our culture changes. They evolve with culture.

Naturally acquired immunity and vaccines have been our most effective defenses against biological viruses. Vaccines safely stimulate an immune response by mimicking the offending microbe with proteins that create a biological recognition and response, but not infection. Awareness of psychic illness can function like a vaccine and help inoculate us against behavior-borne viruses. The tactics employed by psychic illness described in this book are attenuated and neutralized behavior-borne virus, isolated and printed on paper. Sufficient to inform but insufficient to infect, they can provide some measure of inoculation. When people become aware that psychic illness exists, how it works, its limited benefits, its many costs, the existence of a better way to live in the world, and that acting reasonably, responsibly, and treating others with kindness and compassion leads to a better life, then natural consequences come into play and behavior begins to change. It's a better deal. Reward and punishment. Psychic illness is the path of pain and destruction. That lifestyle is a dog.

It is time to reclaim the narrative. We need public discussion about the two paths and strategies for following the better way. We need this represented in news, social media, shows, films, books, and websites. When I was a young man, we called this consciousness raising. Let's begin discussing what is happening now in this context and what we can do about it. We can teach practical skills for identifying inappropriate behavior and dealing with difficult people and trying situations. These can be represented in media and discussed in families and other groups. Are you an academic looking for a new research project? Are you an author or publisher in need of fresh material? Are you looking for a new start-up? Do you work in the media? Are you an influencer or podcaster? Do you write songs? Are you a pastor or a parent? Do you belong to a book club or have friends you talk to? These are universal, unmet needs. There are tremendous opportunities here. We need people working on this. Let's use the enormous power of culture as it was meant: to promote psychic health.

Promote Equality, Opportunity, and Justice

Psychic illness is an inferior strategy that is chosen out of desperation. It thrives in desperation. Let's not make anyone desperate. Free and aware people choose health over sickness and life over death. Unmet needs, a lack of options, and insecurity drive psychic illness. Reduce these, and you suppress the virus. If we want people to turn from harm, we must show them a better way and clear the path to it. We must provide opportunities. Healthy people don't need or want psychic illness. They have alternatives. *More attractive* alternatives. We protect people from pathological influences by providing options, a better way. We must incentivize contribution and cooperation, remove incentives for exploitation, and cease parasitical zero-sum schemes.

Inequality and injustice reward corruption, incentivize unhealthy choices, and encourage pathological problem-solving; they frustrate, weaken, and push people into socially undesirable acts. Evil feeds well in a world of inequality and injustice. This is no way to run a society. Healthy societies provide opportunities, healthy alternatives. Opportunity changes everything. Opportunity instills hope, motivates behavior, and provides a way out of problems. Opportunity rewards healthy choices, promotes economic and social mobility, and suppresses psychic illness.

The quickest way to dig yourself out of a hole is to focus on healthy goals, things you greatly desire, and go after them. For our society to be healthy, people need opportunities to grow. It is very much to our advantage to minimize artificial, arbitrary, systemic, and institutionalized limitations. We should be limited only by our ability and effort. People have instinctual drives to create, produce, and grow. Societies that fail to harness this squander these resources and promote psychic illness. Our social welfare concepts are backward, viewing people as burdens instead of assets: capable individuals eager to contribute. No one should be artificially held back. This is wasteful, and it is wrong. Our table is large; surely there is room for all.

Sell the Good Life

Psychic illness is an inferior strategy chosen out of ignorance and desperation. People do not select inferior strategies when they are aware of and can access better alternatives. We suppress psychic illness by providing a better way and advertising the fact.

When you listen to people's stories day in and day out, patterns emerge. Strategies people use and the results they get. Some strategies work better than others. You hear how people get into trouble, become lost, and get stuck. You also see them grow and free themselves. One path leads to decay and destruction, the other to a better life. There have always been two paths. We are engaged in a struggle that is older than memory, a war that has cut down some of our best and raised up some of our worst. The outcome will decide our future. This is a contest between two ways of thinking and acting, two ideas of the good life, two ways of walking through the world. Your choices will make or destroy you, your loved ones, all that lives. We stand at a crossroads, and choosing our path now is the defining issue of our age. Everything you value hangs in the balance. The stakes could not be higher.

The virtues have protective effects that shield us from harm. Vices ensnare you in parasitism, decay, and destruction. They control, damage, and limit you. Vices do provide some temporary relief and pleasure, and that is their appeal. They are short-term problem-solvers. But, like addictive drugs, vice becomes less effective over time, requiring more and more for less and less effect, and your life becomes increasingly unmanageable. Vices create a classic vicious cycle that amplifies and aggravates problems over time, gradually sucking the life out of you. They begin with pleasure but gradually transition to pain. The path of vice is one of impoverishment and starvation—social, emotional, moral, and spiritual. Vice robs you in every way that a person can be robbed. It hollows you out and transfers control of your mind, emotions, behavior, and soul to the virus. Take the bait, and you will discover too late that you have entered a trap that is fiendishly difficult to escape.

We labor under the illusion that externals—what happens to us—determine our emotions. Get dumped: sad. Win the lottery: happy. Become paralyzed: sad. We believe this because we immediately experience this but fail to recognize *this is only true in the short term*. In the long term, we reliably revert to our set point of happiness, a characteristic level of feeling good or bad. One year after winning the lottery or becoming paralyzed, most people return to their previous level of happiness. Their emotional state is relatively unchanged. So, if winning the lottery or becoming paralyzed doesn't change our long-term happiness, what does?

Our thinking and behavior determine our long-term, characteristic level of happiness. Externals—such as life events, power, money, sex, and status—cannot make you happy. Only your mind and actions can make you happy. Most of your pleasure and pain come from what you think and do, things you can change. Happiness is synthetically manufactured in your mind. It is a chosen interpretation of events. The happiest person I've ever known was a man who had suddenly learned he had just six months to live. I will never forget his words: "You don't see it. *I* didn't see it. *The world is such a beautiful place.* When I heard I had just 180 days to live, all the things I *thought* were problems no longer mattered.

I'm getting everything I can out of each day now." He waded into and befriended a gang of neighborhood toughs and became their valued senior mentor. He made it his mission to teach everyone he met that life is precious. He no longer focused on superficial cares. He focused on what mattered, and the world profoundly changed. Beauty is in the beholder.

I have treated people with disfiguring disorders who were in constant pain. They could not work. They would die early. Half their children would inherit the condition and share their fate. And yet, they were reasonably content. I have also treated people who had decent childhoods and good lives. They were young, healthy, and employed. And yet, they were miserable and dysfunctional, sincerely angry about how life had treated them. There is surprisingly little relationship between externals and happiness. Externals don't matter much. Internals do.

People don't talk about money in therapy. Even when they're homeless, they don't talk about money. They talk about other people. No one has ever told me they want a bigger home, a fatter bank account, more power or status, possessions, or drugs. At our core, we all want the same things. We want love. We want purpose, meaning, connection, stability, health, and peace. We want to care and be cared for. We evolved to want these things because they have survival value. They move us forward and let us last. They *mean* something. What happens to you in life matters less than how you think about it and respond to it. Internals determine happiness, and we can control internals. What we think and do matters. Immensely. More than anything else in life. Be careful what you wish for, what you think and do, the strategies you choose.

If you believe that externals will make you happy, your efforts will focus on externals. You will waste your time avoiding difficult thoughts and responsibilities, life's normal challenges, and your actions will become ineffective, chasing the next quick fix in a doomed attempt at the good life. If you believe that factors beyond your control determine your fate, you make yourself helpless and powerless. You will feel victimized, become a complainer, and may be tempted to control others or vent your frustrations on them. The good news is that your happiness doesn't depend on money, power, status, things going your way, or even good health. Your happiness depends more upon how you use your brain and your body. And these are under your control.

We are born neither good nor evil but with the capacity for both. We live in a time when two very different strategies compete for our selections. When given a choice, most people will meet their needs and solve their problems in healthy ways that affirm life. Life satisfies us. Evil leaves us cold and hungry, starved on empty promises. Evil is a bad deal, an inferior strategy that produces inferior results. People don't typically go down that path without having been seriously spoiled, exploited, neglected, or mistreated. Evil is an attempt to solve problems that reproduces during a struggle to free ourselves from its artificial problems. Evil is not enjoyable. It is an unnatural, man-made, inferior substitute that imprisons us. The evil in this world is what we do to one another. Evil issues from and returns to us. Psychic illness may be a disease, but it is a disease of our own making. Evil requires choice. When we no longer hurt each other, when we no longer feed evil, when we choose to love one another, we will have realized our

purpose in this world. We will have grown and become something more advanced than human beings.

We see before us now a contest between two fundamentally different approaches to life: cooperation vs. exploitation, contribution vs. parasitism, virtue vs. vice. We have the superior product, but we've done a poor job selling it. This must change. We can model, promote, and teach the better way of addressing life's challenges. We can illustrate the different destinations of these greatly divergent paths and the superior rewards of the better way. Psychic illness is all about easy answers, immediate gratification, stealing resources, and concealing and offloading costs. The better way requires effort and time, but it brings the very best that life has to offer. Its rewards increase with time, and life gets better and better. Do you desire happiness and prosperity? This is the path. Love is the better way.

In 1852, Harriet Beecher Stowe published *Uncle Tom's Cabin*, a novel that educated people about the realities of slave life and profoundly affected attitudes toward African Americans and slavery. It sold millions of copies and was instrumental in raising consciousness about the human impact of the corrupt practices of that time.

In 1887, Jacob Riiss published the best-selling book *How the Other Half Lives*, photographic essays that used newly invented flash photography to expose the squalid conditions in New York tenements averaging more than 30 persons per unit. Photographs were in-your-face, emotionally gripping documentation of the horrors of the housing crisis of that day. Riis is credited with stimulating housing reform and helping to launch the Progressive Era.

Today, millions of people are lost and missing out. They are hungry for a better way: a constructive purpose, meaningful activity, clear direction, and badly needed tools and skills for navigating and changing a problematic culture. Are you a writer, musician, playwright, sculptor, painter, photographer, artist, scriptwriter, actor, activist, salesperson, community organizer, educator, healer, programmer, or advertiser? Do you belong to a service organization that needs a worthy cause? Are you a member of the clergy? Do you work with a charitable organization that connects with people in need? We have one of the best products ever created, and you are needed to promote it. We need more people working to build a just and sustainable world and modeling this for others.

Strengthen Existing Defenses Against Psychic Illness

We possess a wide variety of defenses against psychic illness but have neglected many of them. Strengthening these defenses helps to contain it.

We are protected by the social contract. This includes cooperative endeavors such as our values, beliefs, mores, common practices, healthy relationships, social cohesion, institutions, representative government, codified human and animal rights, economic opportunity, and established public services such as education, public welfare measures, health care, and law enforcement. We are protected by sustainable and equitable management of natural and financial resources. Such things promote opportunity and economic security and decrease desperation, limiting psychic

illness. Notions of human dignity, fairness, equality, and social, economic, and political justice are effective antibodies that curtail psychic illness as well. The fact that all these defenses have simultaneously come under attack reveals the work of an external pathogen. BBV is a mind manipulator and destroyer of societies. Your neighbors are not the enemy. Joining together is our path out of this mess.

Science defends against psychic illness. Science is a relatively dispassionate and deliberative process that employs verifiable methods to determine and address reality, making it an effective tool for stripping away static and camouflage and getting to the truth of a thing. To prevent this, psychic illness attacks science and scientists to counter their threat to its operations. It suppresses and distorts scientific research, strives to delegitimize science, and floods culture with baseless, misleading, dishonest, and agenda-driven misinformation and pseudoscience.

Reason and logic reveal irrational thinking and flawed arguments, protecting us from emotional manipulation. Reason and logic help us evaluate the truth of thoughts and ideas and our best course of action. They check falsehoods and foolishness to decrease unwise behavior. We have two main decision-making systems: our head and heart, reason and emotion, our neocortex and limbic system. They evolved at different times, occupy different parts of our brain, follow different rules, and have different strengths and weaknesses. Psychic illness confuses us by provoking primitive base emotions such as anxiety, fear, greed, and anger to bypass the more modern and logical parts of our brain. This makes people easier to manipulate and control.

Representative governments protect us from psychic illness. We left our barbarian ways because civilization was a better deal. The primary function of government has always been to protect us from exploitation and harm. Beware of people who want to weaken and dismantle democratic government. Good government uses rules to equitably regulate minimum standards of behavior and bring relative stability to everyday life. You have an idea of what to expect. You can plan ahead and have some expectation of being treated rationally and justly. Infrastructure is built, laws are enforced, banks are held accountable, and pollution, deforestation, product and workplace safety, employment practices, and food quality are managed. Protections are in place. You can conduct business, travel, and not worry about your kids, parents, future, health, property, or safety so much. You can make and build things without having them taken from you. You have an equal say in choosing the people who make and enforce the law and decide disputes. These are all fruits of representative government that contribute to our freedom. They also greatly interfere with the operations of psychic illness.

Psychic illness attacks the very idea of government. People say, "Government is the problem." No, it is not. Government is the protection. Democratic governments and just laws serve the interests of ordinary people. They standardize procedures, prescribe punishments, and prevent exploitation by the powerful. They protect us from arbitrary rule. The prospect of life without these protections is terrifying. We have been there before, and it was poor, nasty, brutish, and short (Hobbes, 1651/2008). It was so bad that millions of people fought and died to get us out of there.

Talk radio often focuses on second-guessing and picking apart government in the smallest detail. It is unhealthy to make entertainment of criticizing the government. Have you noticed we are not encouraged to make entertainment of criticizing corporations? Why is that? Representative government is a collective endeavor. The virus attacks collective endeavors because they protect and defend us from psychic illness. Cooperative strategies form connections, share resources, and distribute risks. They resist psychic pathology. Psychic illness seeks to dismantle government protections so it can operate unimpeded. It wants you exposed and vulnerable. Representative government is a safeguard against evil. Good government protects rights by balancing your rights with other people's rights. These protections have worked so well for us that they have become somewhat transparent, and we tend to take them for granted now. We have forgotten the horrors of the past.

Do not be so foolish as to let down this shield. If you do this, there will be no returning. Once you cross that line and then learn too late that you made a mistake, there will be no turning back. Once your government has been broken and bad people rule, you will never be allowed to vote them out. Evil does not relinquish power. Evil does not share wealth. If we cross that line, the camouflage will soon be lifted. Too late, you will see raw evil revealed and find yourself staring into the face of a grinning, newly released predator who sees you as nothing more than a naked and defenseless meal.

Democracy defends against psychic illness. Compared to other forms of government, democracies are less warlike and more peaceful. They do a better job of providing for their citizens.

Democracies tend to have higher standards of living. They generally have better education and healthcare systems and tend to promote tolerance. Psychic illness actively undermines democracy by rigging institutions with corrupt financial and political incentives, engaging in partisan redistricting and gerrymandering, imposing unjustly restrictive voter registration and ID laws, closing polling places, purging voter registrations, permitting unrestrained and anonymous political contributions and unrestrained lobbying, advocating for unrepresentative government, co-opting courts, refusing to certify and attempting to overturn elections, attempting insurrection, and installing leaders for life. Baking corruption into institutions bakes evil into society. It enables the corrupt and encourages those who are not corrupt to become corrupt. Psychic illness is the inferior strategy and cannot win an honest, fair fight on the merits. To compensate for this disadvantage, it rigs situations and promotes these underhanded, crooked, unjust, and undemocratic schemes to push its agenda that most people don't want. It steals power and control. It's a thief.

Financial security defends against psychic illness by increasing opportunity and decreasing desperation. When people are financially secure, they have options. They are less likely to turn to pathological problem-solving, and they are more likely to vote. Psychic illness promotes financial insecurity and poverty for these reasons and because the psychically ill enjoy power, inequality, and inflicting pain. This is, after all, a sickness of the soul.

Education suppresses psychic illness and defends against it. Education increases general knowledge, employment options, income, knowledge of alternatives, and political participation, including voting. It makes people aware of and resistant to nonsense. For these reasons, educational disenfranchisement and the promotion of ignorance are common tools of psychic illness used against us. Attacks against intellectuals are also common, as is labeling educated persons "elites." Psychic illness thrives on ignorance. Education is an antidote to ignorance that weakens psychic illness.

Healthcare, including medical and mental health services, defends against psychic illness by reducing stress upon individuals and maintaining their resistance. During the COVID-19 pandemic, efforts to delegitimize medicine increased enormously, and verbal and physical attacks on healthcare providers were commonplace. BBV correctly perceives that functioning public health and health care systems defend against psychic illness. In the past, people were stigmatized for receiving mental health services, discouraging treatment that could reduce their vulnerability to psychic illness. For this reason, the virus seeks to remove and limit access to treatments.

Protecting and helping vulnerable individuals defends against psychic illness. As I write this, people are being arrested in some American cities for feeding the homeless. The stated rationale? Public health. Not eating is indeed one way to avoid tainted food. For thousands of years, people have offered food to strangers in need, and it has universally been seen as a good thing, a virtuous act that brings people together. Every major religion recognizes and lauds this activity. Rome has no business banning loaves and fishes. Cruelty is not an unintended by-product of psychic illness. Cruelty is the point.

Children are defenseless and malleable, future parents with many years and children before them, making them ideal candidates for infection. We are not adequately protecting them, and child abuse remains an enormous problem. Child maltreatment runs unchecked through families and generations like an evil plague, as transmissible as a virulent bacterium or genetic defect. Often committed by people who were neglected and abused, hearing of one person harming another, we should inquire as to who hurt *them*. This cycle is preventable and can be stopped.

Life-supporting beliefs and practices defend against psychic illness and protect us from evil. Life-denying ideology is not about principle, freedom, or belief. It's a pretext for misbehavior, an excuse to exploit and abuse. People crave unneeded money and power because the virus uses inequality to remove checks on its behavior and eliminate the necessity of its host having to act with any shred of humanity towards others. It wants to wield power and inflict widespread misery with impunity. People who crave excess money and power are driven by the virus. Great disparity poisons a society and hastens its demise. Healthy societies place reasonable limits on the amount of money and power people may possess, as they corrupt when excessive.

Root Out Corruption

Capitalism runs on incentives. For capitalism to work properly, to serve us and not the virus, it must reward effort, contribution, and accountability, not dishonesty, greed, and theft. In constructing a complex stratified society with extensive specialization of function and division of labor, we have created niches for the corrupt, the criminal, the conqueror, the polluter, the lazy, manipulative, exploitative, abusive, and predatory—new classes of people feeding off the efforts of others with increasingly ingenious methods while making minimal contributions of their own. We have made human parasites possible (Calvin, 2002). Such people would not have lasted a day in the world of our ancestors, but here they flourish. Corruption rewards bad behavior and feeds psychic illness. Healthy cultures do not reward or promote unhealthy behavior. Our culture is not healthy.

Communications, entertainment, and social media corporations have become enormously influential and are now the world's primary means of cultural transmission, overshadowing and even replacing more traditional institutions, such as the family, that for millennia provided carefully thought-out protection and guidance. The news media have been called the fourth estate, suggesting they check the executive, judiciary, and legislative branches of government. Electronic media have usurped education, religion, and individual discourse (Postman, 1985). They now have prominent roles in child-rearing, socialization, enculturation, education, and role modeling. Jim Morrison observed, "Whoever controls the media controls the mind" (Ismi, 2021). This is not healthy. This change was unsolicited and unplanned, and the incentives and motives of corporations are quite different from those of the families and public institutions they replaced.

Institutions, public and private, can become diseased and corrupted. Their powers can be misused. Institutionalized corruption makes psychic illness systemic, greatly amplifying it. Media, political organizations, and corporations are especially vulnerable to corruption because they exist to generate wealth and power. Many people now avoid the news because they find it too *painful.* Our institutions are now often used to incentivize and promote corruption. Diseased speech and behavior are dangerous and should be discouraged. Advertising and profit introduce bias and have a corrupting influence. Free markets are acceptable for selling many goods and services, but some institutions—such as families, schools, government, and churches—should not be driven by economic profit. Some things we value more than money, and rightly so. It is unwise to base our institutions on monetary gain. Bad things happen.

Many media now act as shills for the wealthy and powerful. They peddle sex, violence, and political poison to distract and addict us and push the agenda of a greedy and powerful few. In the past, more people turned to their church for spiritual guidance and protection. Our society has become more secular. We are exposed to far more depravity than people in the past, primarily through electronic media. How is this affecting our minds? How can we protect ourselves? There are forces at work in the world that do not want these questions asked.

Where dutiful parents once watched over their children to protect them from harm, Madison ad men now scheme to exploit them. When kids kill kids for sneakers, we need to see the other parties to the crime. Driven by commercial advertising, our media have deteriorated into instruments of manipulation, extracting wealth and labor from the consumer through surreptitious and illicit means. They provide instruction disguised as entertainment.

Using greed, fear, and sex to incite artificial reactions for financial and political gain, we are plied with simplistic stereotypes and false narratives, substitutes for reality.

Corrupting influences have even been incorporated into product design. In some cases, cell phone addiction is not an unfortunate side effect but designed into the software. People make money off this. Attention has been monetized and feeds an entire attention economy. It may be tempting to blame tech addiction on the user's choices, but addiction can be an intended effect, the result of cynical and calculating software designed to exploit human needs and psychological vulnerabilities (Bosker, 2016).

The strategy to hijack the brain by activating its reward centers has been called "a race to the bottom of the brain stem" (Ibid.). Our brain's most primitive parts are its most vulnerable. Seizing control and hijacking resources is classic parasite strategy. Our brains have been hacked. Manipulation has been reduced to mathematical formulas as artificial intelligence algorithms learn from experience to better plot against us. Choice has been subverted and reduced to a relic, and the problem increases as technology becomes more immersive. Media are made to change thinking. Synthetic foods are engineered to alter behavior. Video games are designed to addict. Shopping experiences are constructed to provoke consumption. That sinking feeling is your free will being sucked out of you.

New technologies should be adopted carefully and cautiously. We should be especially wary of artificial intelligence due to its exponential and unpredictable advancement. The costs and dangers of new technology are generally not readily apparent. There is a long history of psychic illness discovering and exploiting hidden flaws and opportunities in new technologies and using them against us long before we become aware of the risks. It is realistic and prudent to assume that every invention has concealed costs, and we should immediately investigate what they might be. Better this than perpetual surprise.

Psychic illness sows division and discord to discourage cooperation. It wants us at each other's throats and tearing each other apart, a state of everybody fighting everybody. Divide and conquer. It corrupts institutions, turning our individual interests against one another, placing us in conflict, and polarizing us. People naturally follow incentives and work to maximize their interests. Incentivizing bad behavior corrupts people and turns us against one another. It rewards a few at the expense of the many—a theft that divides and impoverishes us all. Radical corporate capitalism, based on conflict, exploitation, and extraction, threatens our freedom and prosperity. Laws that rely on citizen snitches for enforcement are evil things crafted to divide people. Hitler's Germany encouraged children to inform on their parents. Families were devastated, parents killed, and children orphaned so that others could gain power and control. Is this the path we want to follow? Are we no better than this? Other people are not the enemy. The virus is. Wake up—you are having a bad dream.

Some strategies used against us are quite simple. Make people afraid. Encourage irresponsibility, instant gratification, fault-finding, blame, denial, projection, greed, and anger. Celebrate ignorance. Encourage grievances, anger, and entitlement. Tell people they are victims, that something important is being taken from them. Or just flat-out accuse others of what you are doing (e.g.,

Stop the Steal). Stir people up and encourage acting out. Make antisocial behavior acceptable, excusable, permissible, even admirable. Appeal to base emotions. These tactics undermine the fabric of society, and their end goal is a civil war that benefits only prospective warlords. The true villains in this drama are the purveyors of this infected dreck and those using it to gain power.

We are becoming less free. Corruption is a democracy killer that ignores the needs of citizens and makes government unresponsive. Money and power are now shoveled wholesale into the maws of a few gorged individuals—sucking parasites who have insanely more money than they have earned or could ever need. The evil trinity of corrupted media, radical corporate capitalism, and partisan politics is devouring us. They are good at breaking things down, but they build nothing other than schemes to seize control and extract resources. They are destructors who feed by taking things apart. Is it any wonder that our society has become so torn and divided? This is the plan: divided people are easy to impoverish and control. Breaking things apart makes their resources available for extraction. This path is evil, and it leads straight into Hell.

~ ~ ~

It does not have to end like this. In a world that is increasingly interconnected, altruism, accountability, and responsibility are the only sane and sustainable strategies going forward. We are stronger together. For our culture to be healthy and survive, it must be advantageous to cooperate with one another and disadvantageous to parasitize one another, and this must be readily apparent. We need laws and practices that incentivize healthy, life-promoting behavior and discourage unhealthy, life-denying behavior. This benefits and enriches us all. It is time to unite the human family. Our path lies forward. It requires reformed systems with clear incentives to turn to each other and work together to meet our needs and solve our problems, a responsive society based upon the mutuality of our interests, not domination and control of the many by a diseased few. This will address the problem of psychic illness, vastly improve our quality of life, secure our future, and create a standard of living far beyond anything we have ever known.

Politics determine what is incentivized within a society: where resources are directed, who wins and loses. Societies serving the interests of a limited few siphon off resources, damaging the interests of the majority and the whole of society. Inclusive and equitable political and economic institutions are accountable and responsive to their citizens. They direct resources to where they are most needed, and such societies thrive (Acemoglu & Robinson, 2013). The man-made, politically determined incentives installed into institutions determine a nation's ultimate economic success or lack of it, its prosperity or poverty (Ibid.). Concentrating wealth and power impoverishes nations. Societies that disperse wealth and power, provide equal access to opportunities, and reward effort and innovation prosper (Ibid.). What kind of a society do you want to live in?

Culture is a living river of information and instruction flowing through our minds, media, and institutions. This river has become infested with parasitic ideas and practices. We are being bled to death. We need to clean this river, bolster its immune system, increase its antibodies, and stop the wholesale dumping of toxins and pathogens into it. Our moral development lags our technological development, and this endangers us (Sagan, 1980). We've become too powerful. Forget Mars. Mars isn't going anywhere, and present-day schemes of colonizing Mars and creating an Earth II are an impractical diversion and resource drain. We have work to do here on Earth. First, we get our house in order. *Then* we reach for the stars. This is not a moon shot. This is not a Mars shot. This is a galaxy shot to first make us fit for Earth and, when the time comes, become members of a much larger community.

Technology will not save us; changing our thinking and behavior will. If we are to survive, we must rapidly advance our moral development and make it commensurate with our technological expertise. If we don't protect and defend our culture, we will fall. We don't let people poison our food, water, or air, and we shouldn't permit the parasitic subversion and poisoning of our culture and minds through infected, irresponsible, dishonest, manipulative, and exploitative communications and behavior. Such actions are incompatible with freedom and self-rule. Rights are shields, not swords. They are instruments of protection, not tools of exploitation. Rights only work when they are used properly. Freedom is not a one-way street. When people act irresponsibly and abuse their rights, they violate your rights. Defend your rights by respecting other people's rights. Protect your rights by prohibiting cultural poison, acting responsibly, and holding others to these standards. Freedom is not some fairy gift. Freedom requires responsibility (Stirner, 1936). Freedom costs. Treat others as you want to be treated. Be honest in what you say, accountable for what you do, and expect the same from others.

Most of the world's problems today are external manifestations of problems within the psyche. These are not problems of the world; they are problems of the mind. We have projected our nightmares into waking reality and stumble about like half-conscious zombies, wondering what is wrong with the world. There is nothing wrong with the world. There is something wrong with us, with our minds. We solve these problems by healing the psyche and our culture. This is an opportunity to address our oldest and worst problems. This is an opportunity to grow. When we do this, most of our problems will fade.

Increase Personal Strength and Resistance

People are hungry to take control of their lives and build a better world. They want real, systemic change. The need is there, but it is not being met. This is an enormous untapped resource that can be put to good use and pressed into the service of life, as it was meant. We begin by giving people the tools they need to see through the fog of psychic illness and respond to its many challenges. These include teaching critical thinking and problem-solving, improving coping strategies, and teaching practical skills for responding to psychic illness.

Teach Critical Thinking and Problem-Solving

A growing segment of the population is becoming dangerously delusional, mistaking their self-indulgent conspiratorial and persecution fantasies for reality and using these to justify increasing acts of fascism, including voter suppression, antidemocratic practices, denial of rights, violence, and murder. Psychotic thinking is disconnected from reality. It leads to bad things. It doesn't end well. It also makes behavior ineffective because actual problems are not addressed, and stress is applied to things that are not problems, damaging them. Self-serving fictions end poorly.

Thoughts have emotional consequences. The stories in your head affect your mental health and your behavior. They exert power over you. Beware of the stories you listen to and tell yourself. Grievance-collecting and playing the victim are not the answer. They make it easy for others to control you. They feed your worst thoughts, impair your ability to reason, and they can make you chronically malcontent and depressed. For some, they lead to paranoia and violence. Dispensing with honesty, facts, and logic helps only the virus.

People say, "question authority," to which we might add, "question your thoughts and beliefs." Through confirmation bias, much of what we see is created by our brains and the stories we tell ourselves. Thinking is imperfect and often unreliable. Some of humanity's worst acts are committed by people who have managed to convince themselves of the justness of their actions regardless of reason or evidence. Psychic illness excels at inducing self-deception. We have all kinds of thoughts. Not all of them are true. If we don't question our thoughts, it impairs our functioning and can create injustice for others. When you create injustice for others, you corrupt yourself. Be careful of the thoughts you let run loose inside your head. Emotions often influence thinking without our realizing it, and cognitive biases can distort our view of the world.

Unhealthy emotions can alter our thoughts, beliefs, and behavior. If you experience gratification when causing distress to another person, your mind is infected, and you need to step back.

Error-check your thinking and logically examine the evidence for what you think and believe. Beware of people who encourage anger and fear. If someone tells you to be angry or afraid, if their message is illogical, lacks evidence, or they stand to gain by changing your thinking and behavior, these can be signs they are attempting to manipulate you. Logically evaluate arguments. Be skeptical. Ask questions. Look for alternative explanations.

People can be taught analytical skills and inoculated against misinformation (Roozenbeek and van der Linden, 2019). We can teach logic and critical thinking in every grade. We can promote games that require strategy and teach people how to evaluate an argument's validity and a method's effectiveness. We can show them how to assess the costs, risks, and benefits of various life strategies. We can teach people to become sophisticated consumers of information and media. These skills reduce vulnerability to deception and manipulation. They make choices more informed and based upon verifiable reality rather than distorted spin. They defend us from irrational thinking and pathological instruction, reducing the power of psychic illness.

Improve Coping Strategies

We heal by growing. We grow out of problems and then move on. We are all moving; at one place, trying to get someplace else. We are not sick; we are stuck. Being stuck is not an illness. It is the human condition, and growing is the journey of life. We grow by wrestling with challenges: effort stimulates healing and growth. To increase your physical strength, you might lift weights. To become emotionally stronger, you might step outside your comfort zone and confront irrational fears and insecurities. To increase social skills, you might embark upon a series of increasingly difficult social challenges. To enhance your cognitive abilities, you might choose to engage in a series of increasingly difficult mental tasks; this is the strategy we use for education. To increase your moral development, you might ponder ethical dilemmas, learn about and spend time with people different from yourself, strive to understand other people's perspectives, and examine your thinking and behavior and how they impact other people. Effort stimulates healing and growth. Effort makes you strong and free. This is the better way.

Life unfolds from the choices we make, the paths we choose. Different paths take us to different destinations. Good choices lead to good living. Most human problems result from poor choices, inferior strategies for meeting life's challenges. The most common mistake is over-focusing on the short term and choosing quick and easy fixes that provide immediate rewards with little effort. The "easy path" is actually quite hard. Short-term strategies have all their rewards up front. They are easy and immediately rewarding: no effort or waiting required. Their costs, however, pile up on the back end, slowly revealed over time after you are hooked. This reward schedule makes them seductive, especially when you can externalize costs and pass your problems onto others. Externalization of costs is a form of parasitism.

When we over-focus on short-term results, our quality of life gradually deteriorates and we weaken. We enter a vicious cycle where our thoughts and actions make things worse over time. Unaddressed problems accumulate and more and more of the strategy is required for less and less effect. Avoidance, addiction, control, manipulation, blame, denial, projection, and anger all go from bad to worse. You gradually lose control of your mind, emotions, behavior, and beliefs until you can't *not* do quick-fix strategies. You need them just to function, avoid pain, and feel normal. You become a slave to the virus. Short-term strategies are a bad deal. The only thing going for them is that they are easy and offer quick rewards, but that lasts only a brief time. Good luck with that. Short-term strategies are ineffective and addictive. It's a trap we choose to avoid the heavy lifting of dealing with our issues.

Short-term strategies don't build things. They break things down, feed off the released energy, and use them up. They take viable, functioning units, pull them apart, suck out their resources, and discard the remains as waste. Production halts, and you are left with broken bits of rubble, reminders of what had once been an organic, functioning, self-sustaining whole. This is parasitism, and it's rampant in our society. We were given a garden; we are making a garbage dump. Welcome to that Age of Squander. It doesn't have to be this way.

Long-term, lasting solutions have the opposite reward schedule: costs are on the front end, rewards follow later. Long-term strategies build things. They require effort—investments in your future—but patience and sustained effort yield dividends over time, resulting in a much larger total payout. Do you want to live large? Dig in and do the work, plant and nurture some things, tend to them, be patient and persistent, *then* harvest the rewards. Dividends will come rolling in *for the rest of your life*. As time passes, things keep getting better and easier. Problems are addressed, connections are formed, things are built, and all that effort gradually makes you stronger, smarter, more stable, and even more moral and resistant to psychic illness. This is the good life. Compare this to short-term strategies, where rewards shrink, conditions deteriorate, and options disappear. You are left doing dirty deeds just to avoid the pain when you don't do them—addictive withdrawal. There is no effortless hack, no gimmick, no quick fix to life. Lasting rewards require effort and time, BUT they pay quite well and quite reliably. Good things have up-front costs, but their payoffs can go on forever. This is the better way: do the work, be patient, collect the rewards. There are no shortcuts.

Psychic illness encourages us to shirk responsibility, steal resources, and offload problems onto others. It's an easy, quick-fix strategy that isn't easy and doesn't fix. Beware: it corrupts and enslaves you, drives the wheel around, and makes you the monster in someone else's nightmare.

Our way of life is not working. We can no longer afford vice and tribalism. If we are to survive, we must upgrade to virtue and altruism. This is possible. This is within our grasp. We need to make responsible economies, accountable corporations and governments, and lifestyles purpose-built to harness the power of connection, cooperation, and creation. This will do more than just solve our problems. It will transform us and take us to a better place. *And it will save the world.*

Teach Practical Skills for Responding to Psychic Illness

Recall the four steps of transmission: engage, confuse, weaken, corrupt. See how clear it becomes when laid out in lines of black and white. Dead virus. Dry, crusty, safe to look at, a faint shadow of the live stuff. Evil. Raw, naked, unadorned evil. Notice how simple it looks when you strip it bare and lay it out in the light. It is simple. That's its weakness, one of its weaknesses. It cannot withstand light. Light kills it. We can shine a light on it, make people aware of it, and give them the tools they need to deal with it. Of the four realms of the psyche—behavior, thought, emotion, and belief—psychic illness is least able to engage us through thought. Thought is dispassionate and conscious, leaving little place for a rogue behavior-borne virus to hide.

We can inoculate people against psychic illness. We begin by learning its tactics to better understand our situation, reduce their power over us, and acquire skills for responding to them. We can teach the benefits of healthy lifestyles, the costs of psychic illness, the different life trajectories of the two paths, and how to recognize psychic illness. We can teach and practice skills for responding to difficult people and trying situations: first in structured environments, then in real-life situations. Others can help by observing, giving honest feedback, and suggesting ideas for change and growth. Schools can teach practical problem-solving, social skills, parenting, and financial management skills to make kids stronger, less vulnerable, more independent, and more aware. Encouraging children to read literary fiction helps them develop empathy (Rowe, 2018), theory of mind (Kidd & Castano, 2013), social cognition (Cadwell, 2015), critical thinking (Hollis, 2021), and moral thinking (Ion & Kirsten, 2020). Simple cognitive training can make children resistant to depression (Seligman, Reivich, Jaycox, & Gillham, 1995). We already do many of these things; we just haven't thought of them as inoculation.

We can prepare people for life's problems and teach them practical means for addressing them. Religious instruction, moral education, and spiritual guidance can provide potent antibodies that resist pathological instruction. We can increase kids' resilience by providing intelligently selected, moderate challenges and promoting effortful strategies for responding to life's difficulties. Athletics and adventure sports such as hiking, biking, skateboarding, canoeing, kayaking, caving, and climbing provide excellent resilience training. They teach that growth is fun, and they connect people with nature. Classes in logic, writing, and debate sharpen analytical and verbal skills. Trades, arts, and crafts teach practical skills and provide a sense of one's power. These things make people stronger and increase their resistance to psychic illness.

We need these strategies and skills represented in television, print, film, literature, social media, comics, and video games. We need field manuals, workbooks, and practical guides for responding to difficult people, toxic situations, and the challenges of infectious misbehavior. We need workshops and instructional videos demonstrating these skills. Are you an educator, writer, actor, filmmaker, influencer, pastor, or therapist? Your skills are needed.

~ ~ ~

Outline - How to Decrease and Prevent Psychic Illness

I - CULTURAL CHANGES

1. Disrupt engagement:
   a. Deprive of access to vulnerable persons.
   b. Isolate predators from prey.
   c. Educate and immunize populations.
   d. Identify and respond to maltreatment.
   e. Deprive controlling persons of positions of influence, leadership, wealth, power, and control as they use these to corrupt institutions and infect people.
2. Deprive of habitat and food.
   a. Eliminate poverty, minimize inequality, and limit hate speech.
   b. Monitor and control vectors.
   c. Reduce media attention to misbehavior.
   d. Increase media coverage of prosocial behavior.
   e. Moderate internet content.
3. Enhance population resistance. Beginning in childhood, teach people:
   a. morals, logic, ethics, and responsibility. This can begin with language acquisition, e.g., when children can understand and respond to the word "no." Controlling transmitters who have entered the corruption stage and begun transmitting are seldom interested in morals, ethics, or personal responsibility and may be impervious to such appeals and respond only to self-interest.
   b. scientific literacy.
   c. the benefits of a healthy lifestyle.
   d. how to recognize psychic illness.

e. the costs of psychic illness.
   f. effective strategies and skills for responding to psychic illness.
4. Enhance population resistance by providing:
   a. physical safety.
   b. affordable housing.
   c. access to clean water and nutritious, reasonably priced food.
   d. publicly funded universal health care.
   e. publicly funded higher education.
   f. education, training, careers, and jobs that provide a decent standard of living.
   g. meaningful roles that give belonging and purpose.
   h. freedom from discrimination.
   i. economic, social, and political opportunities.
   j. alternatives to unhealthy behavior.
   k. support for relationships and families of all kinds.
   l. support for individuals' abilities to live independently.
5. Promote healthy institutions:
   a. Root out corruption in institutions, i.e., things that benefit a few but cost the many.
   b. Remove incentives for unhealthy behavior, including exploitation and maltreatment.
   c. Install disincentives for unhealthy behavior, including exploitation and maltreatment.
   d. Install incentives for honest, responsible, respectful, prosocial behavior, fair treatment of others, and constructive and productive activity.
   e. Promote justice throughout society, including political, social, economic, racial, ethnic, gender, and criminal justice.

174 / ENDING EVIL

6. Provide:
   a. representative government, the rule of law, equal protection, due process, fundamental human rights, and freedom from arbitrary limitation.
   b. just and sustainable economic systems.
   c. a criminal justice system that incentivizes appropriate behavior and provides opportunities for education and rehabilitation.
   d. regulated banking and equities markets that disincentivize exploitative and antisocial behavior.
   e. business laws that disincentivize exploitative and antisocial behavior.
   f. restorative and sustainable environmental practices.
   g. ongoing investments in human capital, physical infrastructure, and our living environment to maintain these systems in perpetuity for future generations.

II - CHANGES TO BE MADE BY INDIVIDUALS

1. Modify behavior:
   a. Disengage from unhealthy persons, situations, and activities. Engage with healthy, life-affirming persons, situations, and activities.
   b. Learn to meet your needs in healthy ways.
   c. Practice random acts of kindness. When someone does you a kindness, pay it forward.
   d. Get regular exercise.
   e. Learn a variety of practical skills for responding to psychic illness.

    f. Manage your economy: live simply, limit expenditures, vote with your money, avoid debt when possible, and strive for a positive cash flow.
    g. Strive to make healthy choices.
    h. Strive to be aware of your behavior and its consequences for others as well as for yourself.
2. Improve thinking:
    a. Strengthen your mind. Read daily, engage in challenging mental activities, be a lifelong learner.
    b. Strive to make your thinking reality-oriented, constructive, and productive. Be open to feedback from others.
    c. Actively choose how you interpret events and see what works best.
    d. Become informed about how psychic illness works and learn effective strategies and skills for responding to it.
    e. Maintain mental flexibility: connect with people different from yourself and from backgrounds other than what you have experienced. Consider learning another language (Cipolletti, McFarland, et al., 2016) and the cultural history and customs associated with it. Travel. Organize neighborhood and community potlucks. Volunteer. If you are able, spend time living abroad. Sponsor an international student. Read. Learn new skills. Tutor. Celebrate holidays of other lands. Mentor. Try food that is foreign to you. Learn other people's histories.
3. Improve emotional functioning:
    a. Cultivate healthy relationships.
    b. Meet your reasonable needs and provide healthy outlets for your drives.

      c. Discuss your thoughts and feelings.
      d. Admit to and face dilemmas, unhealthy impulses, and unhealthy practices.
      e. Experiment with change.
      f. Place yourself in challenging situations.
      g. Experiment with different ways of thinking about and responding to emotional conflicts, challenging situations, and difficult people.
4. Examine your beliefs:
      a. Interact with people unlike you and travel when you can; expand your first-hand knowledge of the world.
      b. Regularly examine your thoughts and beliefs and their consequences for yourself and others.
      c. Strive to make healthy choices that promote life.
      d. Shun blame, denial, projection, control, and anger. Replace these with responsibility, radical acceptance, humor, and kindness.

III - INHIBIT THE GROWTH OF PSYCHIC ILLNESS

1. Engage → Disengage. Modify existing relationships and form healthy new relationships.
2. Confuse → Clarify. Learn how psychic illness operates and strategies for effectively responding to it.
3. Weaken → Strengthen. Develop personal abilities and social and economic supports, learn practical skills for responding to psychic illness, and provide healthy outlets.
4. Corrupt → Care. Make healthy choices that support life. Seek mutually beneficial cooperative relationships.

Exploit BBV Vulnerabilities

> Don't fight forces, use them.
>
> —R. Buckminster Fuller

The mask is off, and BBV contains the seeds of its destruction. BBV is vulnerable. Infectious diseases are relatively easy to control because they require access. Prevent access, and transmission stops. BBV is weak. It needs impoverished environments lacking alternatives to develop. BBV must feed. People must choose evil and give themselves over to it. Show them a better way, and it starves. BBV is fallible. It needs stealth and confusion to get past our many defenses and fails when we expose it. BBV is foolish. It causes people to work against their own interests. BBV is unattractive. Naked, unadorned evil is an ugly and repulsive thing. BBV is a bad deal. Evil poisons and degrades those who choose it. It hides from examination because examination reveals its flaws, limitations, and inadequacy as a problem-solving strategy. BBV is exhausting. It devours energy. BBV is unnatural. It requires highly artificial and very specific conditions to exist. BBV is ripe for extinction. It has never lived in a world where people understood it and saw its weaknesses and costs laid bare.

Disrupt the Psychic Illness Cycle

We can use existing epidemiological, public health, and psychological methods to disrupt the psychic illness cycle. To survive, all pathogens must have access to a host, infect a host, persist inside the host, and be transmitted to another host. Pathogens are stopped by preventing exposure, adhesion, invasion, ending persistence (killing the organism or clearing it from the host), or preventing retransmission. Psychic illness is an obligate pathogen—it requires a host to fulfill its life cycle, an extreme adaptation to a host. This dependence upon the host makes obligate pathogens vulnerable, and obligate pathogens are recognized as relatively easy to control using established epidemiological and public health practices.

Parasites and infectious organisms are controlled by depriving them of habitat and access to hosts and reducing risk factors. Psychic illness risk factors include increased exposure and reduced resistance. Decrease people's exposure and increase their resistance, and you suppress the disease. Infection requires environments that provide suitable habitat, access to vectors, and hosts with undeveloped resistance. Making environments hostile to psychic illness, reducing viable vectors, denying access to hosts, and increasing host resistance suppresses BBV.

We increase people's resistance by making them less needy, more aware, and skilled at handling manipulations. Psychologically unhealthy, unsanitary, and corrupted environments with few opportunities facilitate the incubation and transmission of psychic illness, and they can be modified to suppress and defeat the disease.

We have a long history of successfully addressing infectious diseases, and this has provided us with numerous proven epidemiological, public health, and psychological methods to disrupt BBV processes and protect vulnerable people. With effort and ingenuity, these can be adapted to address psychic illness.

Integrate Management of Behavior-Borne Viruses

Identify and Monitor Behavior-Borne Virus Activity. Create working definitions of BBV strains and functional descriptions of their unique actions. Create, implement, and refine systems to identify and monitor behavior-borne viruses, environments that facilitate them, risk factors that promote them, and vectors that carry them.

Adopt Prevention Strategies. Deny BBV access to hosts and vectors. Educate populations and promote healthy practices to enhance population resistance. Develop sanitation practices to reduce exposure. Screen and assess for risk factors and symptoms. Employ case finding, contact tracing, and outbreak management.

Set Action Thresholds. Identify points at which actions are to be taken, e.g., BBV activity and BBV-related adversities (e.g., child abuse, bullying, trauma, abuse of power, crime, assaults, murders, and suicides). Create a menu of responses and protocols that can be implemented when these thresholds are met.

Apply Control Strategies. Provide health education, training, treatment, and rehabilitation for people who request it. Proactively work to monitor and manage public institutions. Forego close-quarter housing in highly infected institutional populations (e.g., prisons and jails).

Make a Science of Behavioral Virology

It is time to begin a coordinated scientific investigation and response to psychic illness. We already study biological virology and electronic virology. It is time to make a science of behavioral virology, map this disease, and develop and implement effective new means of prevention and treatment. The suggested first steps include the following:

1. Assess the hypothesis: "Evil is a disease."
2. Develop tools to detect, characterize, and assess behavior-borne viruses and psychic illness.
3. Develop diagnostic and classification criteria.
4. Inventory, catalog, and categorize BBV variants.
5. Identify and monitor BBV activity.
6. Conduct basic research, including multidisciplinary observation, modeling, experimentation, study, integration, and publication.
7. Determine the frequency (if at all) that BBV arises spontaneously, as opposed to behavioral transmission, and the conditions that facilitate this, e.g., examine the establishment of dominance hierarchies between twins and what happens when single children are indulged, not challenged, and protected from the consequences of their actions.
8. Identify risk factors and protective factors associated with psychic illness.
9. Describe the intervening variables between BBV exposure, infection, and progression to the corruption phase.
10. Document BBV variants, the BBV life cycle, types of hosts, and exploitation of vectors.
11. Develop evidence-based education and prevention programs, skills training, and psychological treatments.
12. Develop model curricula, policies, regulations, laws, and initiatives to address psychic illness.

Vote With Your Money

In *The Wizard of Oz*, Dorothy makes an arduous journey to fulfill the Wizard's seemingly impossible task. It is only after succeeding, and the curtain is pulled back, that she sees the wizard revealed for the humbug that he is and discovers she had the power to get what she needed all along. We are Dorothy. Those ruby slippers? Every time you make a purchase, you vote with your money. You dispense rewards, and rewards influence behavior. Most of us live in some variation of a capitalist system, and flawed as it may be, it does respond to purchases. One percent of the population cannot control ninety-nine percent of the population without their cooperation (Attenborough & Briley, 1982). We are the labor. We are the market. Without us, nothing happens.

Use your power: practice economic non-cooperation and disobedience. Vote with your money and make it count. Boycott products, services, and media that don't align with your values. Do not support corporations with poor human, animal, or environmental practices. Support workers' rights to humane working conditions and fair payment for their labor and products. When you can, buy from small, locally-owned businesses and family-owned farms. Community-supported agriculture provides high-quality, fresh, nutritious food while you connect with the people who grew it. Invest in your community. Do this, and you provide important support to the local economic system you inhabit while enabling viable alternatives to the corporate economy. Producer, consumer, and financial co-operatives and mutuals also provide access to more democratic and locally oriented enterprises.

Want Less, Live More

> A man is rich in proportion to the number of things which he can afford to let alone.
>
> —Henry David Thoreau

Our needs and desires can be used against us. Is this a time of reduced expectations or increased opportunities? We have been sold a lifestyle that is not working for us. Do you yearn to be free? Change your lifestyle. Enjoy the finer things in life. A minimalist lifestyle transforms your situation, decreases consumption, and increases sustainability. It is inexpensive, readily available, and highly adaptable, fulfilling us in ways possessions cannot. It focuses on things that matter. It provides immediate independence, power, pleasure, freedom, and control.

The more we have, the more we want. Nothing is enough, and we are never satisfied. It never ends. I owe, I owe, off to work I go. To get off the buy-borrow-work hamster wheel, you need to know the secret: *once your basic needs are met, you will never be fulfilled, never be made content, by having more.* Never. Look at billionaires. They have, *how* much? And yet, they spend their time and energy trying to *get more*? What is wrong with this picture? You will only be fulfilled by choosing to be satisfied and wanting less. The problem is not that you have too little. The problem is that you desire too much (LaFleur, 1988).

The sellers of the goods and services you buy will never tell you this. They want you working. For them. Endlessly. We imagine that externals will fill the void. Sure, externals feel good for a while, but the hunger always returns, and you want more. More stuff, more money, more attention, more control, blah blah blah, and off you go, hooked. The better way is to enjoy what you have. Savor the moment, relish the experience, seize the day. No thing can compare. A wise man once spent two years on the edge of a pond and unlocked the universe. This is a treasure hunt: go find him.

Invest in People

A society is poorer for every person it holds back and locks out. People are assets, and investing in them returns dividends. It improves our quality of life, makes us strong, and increases resistance to psychic illness. Opportunity is protective. When a better way is available, people are less likely to choose the path of pain. This is not where we are now.

In the United States, 40 years of flat wages and increasing costs have benefitted a prosperous minority and squeezed out the majority. Unfortunately, many voters haven't yet made the connection between massive wealth transfer and their economic plight (search "supply-side economics" and "trickle-down economics" for the interesting history of this heist), and conservative media have successfully diverted their distress into anger—not at the cause of their plight, but at liberals. That's some trick. Rip someone off and then convince them to blame the guy who tried to stop it. This is classic psychic illness: create a problem, prevent its resolution, then feed off the extracted resources while blaming others.

If you want to know where your money went, look at who has the money. It sure isn't liberals. Nobody "earns" a billion dollars.

A greedy and privileged few sit red-handed on mountains of cash while shamelessly rigging once-democratic systems in their favor, and you think *liberals* are to blame? Liberal democracy is about sharing. It's about fairness. It's about inclusion and justice. These are good things. They benefit you and your children. If you are looking for someone to blame, liberals and Democrats are far from perfect, but—you've got the wrong guy.

Greed creates a defect of empathy, and people become numb to others' suffering. Greedy people don't care about other people. They care about money and power. *Other people's* money and power. If you haven't noticed, we are not sitting at the table. Psychic illness manipulates and divides us to seize control and steal our wealth and power. It distracts us with fake, made-up claims and phony issues to make us emotional, so we don't see the real villain, don't see what is ripping us off. This is what thieves do. We are being treated like marks, and it's working.

It doesn't end here. The goal of BBV is to break the government and crash the economy. It uses economic pain strategically as a softening-up maneuver. For the wicked, pain is a good idea, a useful tool to break people down. Psychic illness uses conflict and stress to make people distracted, needy, vulnerable, afraid, angry, and outraged, ready to morph into something else. It wants zombies—unthinking, unquestioning, obedient minions. Desperate people do desperate things. They act irrationally and settle for things they wouldn't consider in better times. Emotional people can be manipulated and controlled. Scoundrels do this and then blame others, subterfuge to put us off their scent and mislead us. These people are just getting started. When they have us where they want us, when we finally realize that we've been taken, when it becomes painfully evident that this was the plan all along, it will be too late to do anything about it.

For the past 42 years, *for two long generations*, the United States has embarked on a massive conservative experiment. Supply-side, trickle-down economics radically restructured the economy, systematically transferring money from those less well-off to the wealthy. It didn't work. It failed spectacularly, and it is tearing America apart. The Great Siphoning succeeded only at what it was intended to do all along: take money from those who earned it and give it to those who don't need it. What a terrible idea. We keep this up, and the United States defaults on its debt, we go into a depression, the world goes off the dollar standard, and we lose our ability to borrow our way out of a depression as we did in the past. This is a trap. There will be no way out. Economic and political power will be consolidated into a single, brutal entity, efficiently maintained through control of modern media and surveillance technology. All the pieces are in place. If we fail this test, we risk falling into a black hole of totalitarian fascism from which there may be no escape, a permanent end to human self-rule. There will be no freedom, only power and control. Evil does not share power (Jackson, 2001). Evil does not relinquish control. Evil is insatiable. It stops only when overpowered by force or when it starves, often after killing its host.

How can I predict this? If you see a person falling through the sky without a parachute, you know their trajectory and inertia will remain unchanged, and they will die. It's simple math. When you see a vicious cycle unfolding with powerful forces in play, without sufficient arresting counterforces correctly placed and applied, you can be confident that the process will play out to the end. We are trapped in a chain reaction of psychopathology stuck in a self-reinforcing positive feedback loop. Vicious cycles maintain their direction and momentum until they are arrested by countervailing forces or undergo systemic failure and collapse. Simple extrapolation of current events—substantiated by the many confirmatory warning signs now presenting as we travel down this path—tells us where we are being led. The actions of psychic illness are predictable, played out like a chess game. If you know the board and have studied the players, you can induce strategy from tactics and predict moves ahead. First, they position their pieces, and then they strike. Thinking strategically is how chess games are won. Acting strategically produces tells that signal intention. We are being treated like cattle, and that large man standing at the top of the ramp wearing a leather apron and holding a sledgehammer is not your friend.

When you extrapolate the conservative agenda and actions of the past 40 years, this is where we are headed. This is where their leaders want us. If you think things are bad now, you have no idea where they are taking us. This garbage is straight out of the dictator's playbook. It always ends in disaster. It never ends well. Hitler left sixty million dead, six million incinerated, and his country in rubble. He was stopped only because external forces were able to effectively organize and oppose him. There are no equivalent external forces in the world today. No cavalry is going to come to save us. We must self-arrest. History is rife with this story, repeated over and over. Hitler was not an anomaly. Hitler was a type, and lessons are repeated until they are learned (Carter-Scott, 1998). Do we really need to go there again to see how this ends? These politicians and media magnates are people you do not want to follow. This is not a road you want to go down. These people care only about themselves. They are using us, and they have big plans for us. Beware. Do not feed their illness. Do not give them money. Do not give them votes. Invest in yourself, your family, your neighbors, your country, your planet, and your future. Invest in things that matter, not some greedy, power-hungry, infected fools. Do not follow the diseased. It ends badly.

History is clear on this: when countries invest in their people, everyone thrives. The best place to put money and resources is where they are most needed. Putting money and resources where they are needed makes economic systems responsive, accountable, and prosperous. It is time to return to demand-side, Keynesian economics and shift taxes back to where they were the last time we prospered—more on the wealthy. This puts more money in people's hands, which increases spending on goods and services and stimulates the economy. *Put money and resources where they are needed, and good things happen.* Put money into the hands of people who need it, and it changes hands far more quickly than giving it to the wealthy. We know this works. We did this from 1946 to 1976, and it created enormous prosperity. America thrived. America prospered. This was also how we dug ourselves out of the Great Depression of the 1930s.

Demand-side economics was an enormous success. That prosperity was slowly strangled beginning in the 1980s by our transition to supply-side, trickle-down economics, initiating the Great

Siphoning and the unfolding disaster around us today. And yet, policies of transferring even more wealth and power to the wealthy and powerful remain the platform of conservatism. More tax breaks for the wealthy, voter suppression, and power for the powerful is not a good idea. Enough is enough, and more is too much. It is time to change course and put us on a different path.

Going forward, we need progressive tax reform and publicly funded healthcare and higher education. A guaranteed basic income would also be a good start. Transitioning to a green, service-based economy is absolutely essential if we are to maintain anything like our present standard of living. The beautiful thing about investments is that they pay dividends. They give back. Human investments increase our standard of living. They always have. If you seek proof, look at other developed countries. The United States has fallen behind and become the world's first poor rich country. When countries don't invest in their people, everyone loses. There are real-world consequences to bad choices and bad behavior that no spin, ideology, propaganda, lies, or delusional thinking can fix. You are hard-up now because the economic policies of the past 40 years invested in billionaires, not you. Look who benefitted. Look who lost. There's your answer, right in front of you, on the home page of every news outlet.

We have everything we need to solve most of the world's problems. When we unite and pull together, there is nothing we cannot do. This is no time for dog-eat-dog stick your hand in someone else's pocket. This is a time to invest in *us*. This is no time for half measures. This is a time to think big, reach up, and take life to a new level, to build a prosperous, just, and sustainable world. This is a time to do more than solve our problems. This is a time to reach for more and make the world better than it has ever been. We have serious problems, and we need serious people who are ready to address these problems (Reiner & Sorkin, 1995). We don't want the past. We want better. We want more. We want a thriving world where people work together and live in peace. This is not too much to ask. It is time to find our voice and begin the work so plainly laid before us. This is good work. It will change the world, and it will change us.

Reform the Economy

There is not one capitalism; there are many. An incomplete list of its many variations includes advanced capitalism, corporate capitalism, finance capitalism, free market/*laissez-faire* capitalism, mercantile capitalism, oligarchic capitalism, social capitalism, state capitalism, and welfare capitalism (the Nordic model). For over forty years now, under the pretext of supply-side economics, the United States has transitioned to a radical form of corporate capitalism, subordinating democratic government to large corporations and the global financial system. President Eisenhower, a Republican, warned against this in his farewell address to the American people (1961):

> In the councils of government, we must guard against the acquisition of unwarranted influence, whether sought or unsought, by the military-industrial complex. The potential for the disastrous rise of misplaced power exists and will persist. We must

never let the weight of this combination endanger our liberties or democratic processes. We should take nothing for granted. Only an alert and knowledgeable citizenry can compel the proper meshing of the huge industrial and military machinery of defense with our peaceful methods and goals, so that security and liberty may prosper together ... As we peer into society's future, we—you and I, and our government—must avoid the impulse to live only for today, plundering, for our own ease and convenience, the precious resources of tomorrow. We cannot mortgage the material assets of our grandchildren without risking the loss also of their political and spiritual heritage. We want democracy to survive for all generations to come, not to become the insolvent phantom of tomorrow.

—Dwight David Eisenhower

The government that the American people have now is not what they had 50 years ago. It's not what they voted for, and it's not what they want. A coup is taking place, and our government is being overthrown. Psychic illness has metastasized, invaded our institutions, and force-fed us a perverted form of radical corporate capitalism. In this winner-take-all scheme, many large corporations now act as enormous parasites, plundering public resources for private profit while externalizing costs. This is parasitism. Psychic illness has taken up residence in large corporations and banks. Many are infected. Minority wealth and power are on the rise; majority rule and democracy are on the wane. Seizing control and stealing resources is what parasites do. Private corporations feed on public resources and externalize their costs (waste products) back to the public domain. Because radical corporate capitalism is separate from the systems it eats and defecates on, it does not respond to feedback from those systems. With no stake in their health, it has no stop switch. Psychic illness feeds until nothing is left, then licks the plate clean. The Great Siphoning was only the beginning, and the virus is just getting started. Its plan is to scour the planet until nothing is left, to feed until civilization ends, humanity fails, and we go extinct.

American capitalism is brutal now, but it wasn't always this way. Corporations in the United States began as bit players in the economy, insignificant and temporary entities chartered by states for specific, limited purposes and finite periods. They had expiry dates. In the United States, "corporation" is the technical term for a limited liability company. A corporation is a legal fiction designed to limit the responsibility and accountability of the individuals who own it. Stockholders are not personally responsible for the actions of the corporations they create and control. Dr. Frankenstein is free to create monsters, risking only his invested funds. The U.S. Supreme Court has ruled that corporations can even be treated as people with personal rights. Corporate owners have fewer responsibilities; the persons impacted by corporations have fewer rights. I think you see where this is going. During the past 150 years, the role and power of corporations have radically expanded while government protections and corporate taxes have greatly diminished. This is a grab. Effective corporate taxes in the United States had been declining since the 1940s when, in 2017, Congress passed the Tax Cuts and Jobs Act (TCJA), permanently lowering the top statutory corporate tax rate from 35 percent to 21 percent (Floyd, 2023). The TCJA also ended benefits to individuals and families beginning in 2025 (Ibid.). The privately held corporation has become the most powerful institution in the world, and this has caused one disaster after another. With fewer people making decisions, mandated self-interest, reduced accountability of those in power, and reduced protections for citizens, mismanagement and abuse are the inevitable, intended results. This is corruption by design. The majority now suffer so that a minority can party. The Magna Carta, the Renaissance, the Enlightenment, the countless wars for independence and freedom we fought over the past eight centuries—it's like they never happened. We have new masters now.

Our institutions should not function as parasites. We created institutions, and institutions should serve us, not the virus. Franklin Roosevelt defined fascism as the "growth of private power to a point where it becomes stronger than the democratic state itself... ownership of government by an individual, by a group, or by any other controlling private power" (Time, 1938). This is also a good description of institutionalized psychic illness. America is moving toward fascism, driven by psychic illness. The virus is sitting down to feed, and it is just getting started.

Psychic illness is all about the diversion and misappropriation of resources. After 40 years spent listening to people tell their stories, my sense is that these problems have greatly increased. The broader problem is rigged systems that favor psychic illness. You take this same problem, apply it to all our institutions, and you have an existential crisis. This is not sustainable. This is not the stuff of which futures are made. Many of our institutions are failing now because they are not serving us. They are serving the virus.

Conservatives claim that government is the problem, and they offer radical corporate capitalism as the solution. However, for two generations now, conservatives have had their way. Corporate power has greatly increased while government has greatly decreased. Things have not gone well. Protections have been removed, wealth and power have been siphoned, and 90% of workers have watched their income stagnate or decline for 30 years (Stiglitz, 2019), even though their productivity doubled. Our prospects now are less than our parents, and hope of affordable education, steady employment, increasing income, and home ownership is fading. Bankruptcy, addiction, illness, and homelessness are now our concerns. We live in a time of diminished expectations. America is simply not providing for its people the way it did before this conservative experiment began. The radical conservative agenda has been thoroughly tried and thoroughly failed. The radical model of corporate capitalism has succeeded only in benefitting the wealthy at the expense of most Americans while achieving "the highest level of inequality among advanced countries and one of the lowest levels of opportunity" (Ibid.).

Radical corporate capitalism is rigged, reducing competition and incentives while offloading costs to those less well-off and transferring productivity gains to the wealthy. We have socialism for the rich and capitalism for the poor, as large corporations are over-subsidized and under-taxed. Corrupt political systems and unrestrained capitalism incentivize unhealthy behavior and feed psychic illness. The resulting economic and political inequality is destroying representative government. A coup is taking place, and making matters worse, the problems are being blamed on those most impacted while the perpetrators continue to carve up and feed on the carcass of a struggling America.

Follow the money. During the past 30 years, the U.S. economy doubled while inflation-adjusted wages for most people did not budge. Where did all that money go? Follow the money. Worker productivity and corporate profits have soared to all-time highs while labor's share of the GDP is at all-time lows. Follow the money. Possession of stolen property is evidence of theft. We've been robbed by a greedy and privileged few who use large corporations and banks as their bagmen. The über rich sit on more money than they know what to do with. They distract us from their crimes and scheme to steal more by demonizing immigrants, the poor, people of color, LGBTQs, government, and Democrats, spreading outlandish conspiracy theories to take the focus off their behavior. If you want to understand who robbed you and how they did it, follow the money. The preposterous lies they feed you and their attacks on innocent people to put you off their scent are further evidence of their crimes. Follow the money. Their money, *which you earned*, has been used to twist public opinion, change laws, and further rig the system in their favor. It's class warfare, and we're on the losing end. The greedy have fattened up while regular people are headed for slaughter. Excess wealth + disproportionate political power = a self-reinforcing vicious cycle of corruption. This is not democracy. This is plutocracy, a society controlled by great wealth. Plutocracy is incompatible with democracy, and it is driving us to fascism. These people are taking America *down*. They don't want freedom or democracy; they want power and control. Seizing control and stealing resources is what viruses do.

The fascist strategy to gain power is to break the government, crash the economy, and make people desperate. Psychic illness thrives in broken systems and desperate circumstances. Broken systems and desperate people are easy to manipulate and control. They are malleable. This is a classic softening-up maneuver: hit someone on the head to stun, confuse, weaken, and disable them, then move in and have your way with them unimpeded. These people are not your friends. They want your money, freedom, government, and country, and they will say and do anything to take them from you. They are infected, and they want your resources. They will suck out your very souls if you let them. They attack and weaken government because representative government is an effective impediment to evildoing. No government is perfect, but representative government is an ancient protector of rights and liberties. Representative government is one of our best defenses against evil. A world without representative governments is a place where individuals can be stripped clean, made naked and defenseless to predators—raw prey. It is not a world of freedom; it is a world of predation, terror, and slavery. We have been there before, and these people are setting us up and moving in for the kill.

Radical conservatives claim this is about freedom—a clever half-truth that is half-right. Unrestrained capitalism and suspension of democracy and individual liberties are about *their* freedom—to do what they want without restriction. The only freedom the virus values is its freedom to do as it pleases without being limited by the rights of others. The "freedom" it seeks is to pillage, plunder, and feed on people unimpeded. Calling this freedom is a lie. Radical corporate capitalism long ago abandoned free markets and now seeks to rig elections,[3] courts, legislatures, laws, regulations, appointments, foreign policy, trade, banks, taxes, media, markets, and minds in any way it can. The fix is in. Our present brand of capitalism may be many things, but it is not free. It is incredibly costly, the most expensive thing humankind has ever been saddled with. This is not freedom; this is corruption. I say this to radical corporate capitalists: "I believe in competition and free markets. The question is, *why don't you?*" The current conservative agenda (it was not always this way—these people are radicals) is not about freedom and competition. It is about power and control: the power of the wealthy and powerful to do as they wish without restraint by stripping people of the rights that our ancestors fought and died for. *Fought and died for.* All those boys on all those beaches died to fight against fascism, not to adopt it.

Radical corporate capitalism champions a world where power, wealth, and control are held by a private few. The "freedom" of the wealthy and many large corporations is being purchased with our ancestor's centuries-long sacrifices and your impoverishment and

---

[3] For example, Efforts to invalidate and overturn the 2020 presidential election, promote and support violent insurrection, practice partisan redistricting and gerrymandering, limit voter registration, institute restrictive voter ID laws, close polling places, purge voter registrations, disenfranchise voters, allow unrestrained political contribution and unrestrained lobbying are evidence of institutionalized corruption. Such tactics are more often seen in authoritarian regimes than in democracies. They are evidence that psychic illness is tugging us away from democracy and toward fascism. Fascism is attractive to psychic illness because it removes democratic constraints, allowing unrestrained feeding.

thrall. Public wealth and power are channeled wholesale into private hands, creating lost commons and neutered governments. No vote was taken while corporations became our best-funded and dominant institutions, surpassing even the government. And yet, privileged people and large corporations continue to criticize and attack the government and demand even more power and more wealth. Their appetite is insatiable because it is not based on need. It is based on addiction. It is based on infection. They will never be satisfied. Whatever you have, they want. Whatever they have, they want more. The virus drives their behavior. They are possessed. Not by demons, but by a curse older than history.

Government is not the problem. Government is the protection. Wealth and power that were once a public trust established for the benefit of society are now held in private hands for the benefit of a few. This enormous transfer of wealth and power, this ferocious engine of inequality, occurred under the charade of free enterprise and free markets. We've been sold poverty and servitude as wealth and freedom. The private sector now concentrates wealth and power to such an extent that large corporations resemble centrally planned, state-run economies. The problem is not just government versus private ownership; the problem is also the inferior organization and mismanagement that inevitably results from concentrated cores of decision-making and control. Centrally planned economies and enormous uncompetitive corporations harm the public interest. They don't function well. Although we associate these entities with different ends of the political spectrum (socialism and radical corporate capitalism), they both concentrate functions that are better performed by numerous co-equal actors.

No natural system on Earth concentrates resources and control like this. This is unnatural and suboptimal, an inferior way to operate a society.

Democratic governments distribute decision-making to numerous co-equal actors, improving decision-making, increasing stability, and suppressing psychic illness. Concentrated power lacks diverse membership and diffuse decision-making. It dominates, deceives, restricts competition, inefficiently allocates resources, and yields unresponsive, unaccountable, poorly regulated systems that cater to special interests. It devours public resources to benefit a privileged few and externalizes costs to the broader society—a public subsidy of private profit. Concentrated power manufactures poverty. The world does not need government or corporate monoliths. It needs level playing fields filled with numerous and diverse competitors, cooperators, and voters. It needs safeguards and protection from wrongdoing. Concentrated wealth and power are bad economics and poor policy. They put money and resources where they do the most harm and eject their byproducts as waste into the public domain. And they feed the virus.

Corporations are mandated by law to further the interests of their shareholders and place profit above all else. (Bakan, 2004). Environmental, social, and moral concerns are simply not a factor until they risk negative publicity or running afoul of the law and interfering with profit. Even then, insubstantial fines can make unlawful practices profitable. Corporations are legally construed to be persons. If these are persons, they are psychopaths (Ibid.). Corporations are rapacious, and no profit is ever enough. When an entity extracts resources and serves itself to the detriment of others, it is a parasite. An alternative approach is the triple bottom line, where three considerations prevail: people, profit, and planet (Elkington, 1998). We need to base our economies less on competitive extraction and consumption and more on cooperative creation and service. Concentrated wealth and power are not solutions to our problems. Concentrated wealth and power *are* the problem. This is not a time to double down on corporate tyranny. This is a time to reform our economy and government, institute progressive tax reform, adequately fund government services and programs, strengthen regulatory protections, and transition to a more responsible and humane economy.

Capitalism needs regulation. Capitalism needs supervision. Capitalism needs an adult in the room. We need government by the people for the people. We need truly representative government, majority rule, progressive taxation, universal health care and higher education, equality, opportunity, living wages, environmental restoration and protection, freedom to choose, rights to organize labor, and safe living and working conditions. We need protection from dangerous products, humane treatment of animals, replacement of the Electoral College with the popular vote, Senate reform, Supreme Court expansion, and many other progressive changes that will do the greatest good for the greatest number of people. Our economy and government must stop serving the virus. Their mandate is to serve the people. When we followed these strategies in the past, America prospered. We stopped following them, and America declined. Figure it out.

A society's greatest assets are its people and its culture. Cultures can be properly cared for and prosper, or they can be mismanaged and become diseased and rotten. Rotten things die. Cultures dramatically impact every aspect of life. When cultures go down, they take everything with them.

Our current mental health and homelessness crises are fed by a ruthlessly extractive economy, inequality, and lack of representation in government. We've made life unnecessarily difficult for many people, so of course they have problems. The opioid epidemic, now killing over 100,000 Americans per year, has been fed by childhood trauma (Maté, 2018), economic inequality, poverty, insufficiently regulated pharmaceuticals, and inadequate mental health and addiction treatment services. Failure to obey the wishes of most Americans and enact effective gun control legislation (Gallup, 2023) has contributed to an unending series of mass shootings. Cultures are living things that need protection and care. Unprotected and neglected cultures become infected, sick, and die. Their societies collapse. Cultures that are properly cared for and follow nature's laws of survival thrive. Understanding this yields powerful strategies to improve virtually every facet of life, not just for humans but for all that lives.

Our culture is not conforming to the laws of nature. It is not sustainable, and radical corporate capitalism is fundamentally failing us. Most people now struggle to survive while providing unprecedented wealth for a diseased few. Crony capitalism is destroying America. We worship wealth, and it will be the death of us. Our culture is abuzz with parasites feeding faster and faster while taking us down. Psychic illness is adapting, spreading, and killing us. We have the ability to stop, heal, and prevent this, but do we have the will? The path of easy is a short path, and it never ends well.

Our culture has changed us, wiring us for narcissism, greed, consumption, power, and control. We are living below our potential. Cultures are highly programmable and can be rapidly modified. We need to remove incentives for unhealthy behavior and increase incentives for healthy behavior. We need to prevent manipulations of our economy and government, curb lobbying and excessive campaign contributions, enact progressive tax reform, pass financial regulations that protect people from economic parasites, and amend our constitution to make government more representative. It is time to become accountable and empathic, do the heavy lifting that is sorely needed, make responsible choices, and stand with one another. We are better than this. Let's change our culture and wire us for other things. Let's grow.

The path to a better world is clear and attainable if we make responsible choices and stop feeding evil. Let's tax the rich and bring back democracy, effective government, and a just economy. We know this works. We did this in the past, and we thrived. Radical corporate capitalism actively enslaves us. Stop with the lame conspiracy theories, lies, thievery, hate, and anger. They get us nowhere. Don't demonize people who are different from you. Lift them up, and you will be elevated. Don't attack the vulnerable. Defend them, and you will be empowered. Don't hate the poor. Love them, and you will be enriched. This is not complicated: we are stronger together. Our path is clear, and it is a noble path. A better way beckons.

Restore and Protect Our Natural Environment

It is easy to take something for granted when it self-repairs. The living systems we inherited came with incredible resilience and abilities to heal. For most of our time, our technologies were insufficiently advanced to make much of an impact, and we could act without regard for the consequences of our actions. That time is gone. We are too many now, our technologies too powerful. A great adjustment has begun. People die, ecosystems fail, species perish, and resources dwindle. Our options are narrowing. To survive, we must transition from consumption and growth-based economies to service and maintenance-based economies. This is our only path to survival.

We have changed from hunting and gathering to shopping and hoarding. Leisure has become synonymous with distraction. Our lives have become this empty and shallow. We need meaning. We need purpose. We need connection. Our economies, based on production and consumption, must change and become based on service. We need to move from objects to activities, to lives concerned not with extracting, acquiring, and consuming more but with living, doing, and being more (Fromm, 1976). Art, education, health care, religion, music, recreation, cultural exchange, world peace, basic scientific research, innovation and invention, athletics, leisure, public service, and social interaction—the most interesting, rewarding, and desirable activities of humankind—can all flourish with minimal impact on the biosphere. We need to move from a consumption and waste economy to a service, experience, and recycle economy, to manufacture items designed to be returned and reused. The opportunities are enormous, not just to overcome our worst problems, repair and improve the economy, but to grow as human beings, become truly civilized, and greatly improve our quality of life.

Psychic illness is the wrongful control and exploitation of other life. Not just humans but all that lives (Fouts, Mills, & Routs, 1997). Values nudge us away from such acts, for experience proves them unhealthy. But now, we gnaw, suck, and tear away at the very ground beneath our feet, extracting the last measure of vital essence for monetary gain. If evil is satisfying one person's desires at the expense of other people's needs, then our extraction of every last resource from the Earth to support exorbitant and unsustainable lifestyles at the expense of all future life is patently evil. We have surpassed the carrying capacity of this planet and are now devouring our future even as we rush toward our own destruction. And for what? For a few trinkets, status symbols, transitory gadgets, fleeting pleasures, more possessions than we even know what to do with. While people starve and species vanish. We are not meeting needs; we are gorging appetites. We don't need more things; we need better lives. From this point on, we improve our lives not by possessing or consuming more but by learning, living, loving, giving, and being more. We need to make pollution costly and environmental restoration profitable, embrace low-impact lifestyles, stop externalizing costs, and make an item's purchase price reflect its true costs—including its social and environmental impact (Hawken, 2010). We can do this not with moral mandates but with self-organizing market principles that correctly use economic incentives that reflect the true costs of one's actions (Ibid.).

We have conquered hunger, but can we conquer desire? We worship wealth at the expense of our physical, mental, emotional, and spiritual well-being (Fromm, 1976). Life is sacred. Life is holy. What we are doing to life on this planet is wrong. Our living environment crumbles beneath us as we chase the good life, which we presently seem to define as more money and power. This cannot last. Many of today's myths are pretexts for an underlying materialism that is eroding our quality of life (Veblen, 1899/1994). Freedom from want does not provide freedom from fear. Once your basic needs are met, quality of life comes not from possession; it comes from action (Fromm, 1976).

Consumption-based lifestyles are driven by artificial desires that are largely unrelated to needs. Consumerism spurs us to endless acquisition, slavishly driving the rich man's economy. A typical home today provides better living conditions than those of emperors and kings of the past. Insatiable appetites come not from need but addiction, self-reinforcing feedback loops. The more you have, the more you want. *It* will never be enough until *you* are enough. If you can never be satisfied, you become a slave to your appetites and enjoy nothing. We have been taken from ourselves and estranged from each other. Our technologies have become so powerful that consumption-based lifestyles are consuming the planet and destroying species at an exponential rate. This path is taking you to a place you really don't want to go.

Biology and culture run on different clocks, and we pursue short-term interests at the peril of our long-term survival. That long-term is now shrinking, staring us in the face and licking its lips as we rush blindly toward its devouring jaws. We have contaminated all of Earth's organic matter—vegetation, bone, shell, and living tissue—with radiocarbon from nuclear explosions (Sakharov, 1958/1990). We alter the world for our transitory comfort, destroying habitat, eradicating species, and destabilizing ecosystems by reducing their complexity. This cannot last. We are poisoning our only planet and plundering your children's heritage. We are losing life-sustaining diversity at an astonishing rate. We are killing the world that sustains us, the Earth that gives us life, that *is* life. Have we really come so far? Even our chimp cousins have sense enough not to soil their nests. There is a better way: We change the world by changing how we see the world.

Chapter 5

CROSSROADS

Humankind is at a crossroads. We have not faced decisions of such consequence since we began manufacturing stone tools and emerged to consciousness 2.6 million years ago. It now seems that everything that came before was preparation for our decisions of the next 100 years. School is out. Playtime is over. Aware and free and immensely powerful, human beings are loose upon the world. Now we have freedom. Now we have choice. Let us use these things wisely and for the benefit of all.

There are two paths before us now, and so has it always been. The path of light and the path of darkness. Growth and decay. We inhabit a knife's edge. The virus would have us choose the lower path, even as we are beckoned to a higher calling. There is goodness in this world, things worth fighting for (Jackson, 2002).

There is a story going around now that white people are exceptional, entitled, oppressed, and discriminated against by the poor and non-whites; that the wealthy and privileged few are clever, deserving, and estimable while the poor and marginalized are lazy and parasitical; that collective endeavors such as a middle class, equality, representative government, personal responsibility and accountability, civility, respect for human rights, tolerance, kindness, compassion, cooperation, and sharing are inferior to tribalism; and that this story leads to an exalted state where the wicked are punished, the fit prevail as ordained by God, and this path magically attracts wealth.

There is another story, a story of a world that has lost its way during a time of great change, a world that has unnaturally concentrated wealth and power into fewer and fewer hands, causing a rapid and dramatic decline for most of humanity and all of Earth's living systems. This is a story of a small minority, an increasingly privileged few who use crass appeals to greed, fear, and anger to squeeze the remaining life out of the many for no purpose other than to further their own addictive enrichment and evil gratification at the suffering of others. It is a story of our kind teetering on the edge of a great cliff, ready to plunge into the dark pit, or shake off this nightmare, spread our wings, and soar.

These stories live within each of us, and your life moves in the direction of your strongest story (Groeschel, 2021). Your choice now is, what story will you listen to and tell yourself? You stand on this precipice, one voice whispering in your ear, stoking your primitive emotions and tempting you down the short path, telling you to trust without thinking and leap without looking. But from every heart, and surely from God above, comes the other voice and the other story. This voice and this story engage your mind as well as your emotions; your conscience as well as your appetites; your soul as well as your desires. The question before you now is, what is your strongest story? What voice will you heed? What path will you follow? Will you fall, or will you fly?

Love Wins

> Love is wise; hatred is foolish. In this world, which is getting more and more closely interconnected, we have to learn to tolerate each other and learn to put up with the fact that some people say things that we don't like. We can only live together in that way. If we are to live together and not die together, we must learn the kind of charity and tolerance which is absolutely vital to the continuation of human life on this planet.
> —Bertrand Russell (1959)

There is hope. The thing about hardship is that it can break you down or build you up. It depends upon how you respond to it. Stress and choice change things, and our hearts and souls are being tested. We can make ourselves into monsters, or we can grow and become better. For good or ill, the wheel is in spin, and there is no telling how this will end.

Pain is a needed and valuable signal. It draws our attention to problems and motivates us to do something about them. Pain and problems are opportunities, chances to improve our lives. This is good medicine. Greed hungers for gratitude. Harm cries for healing. We can use these problems to our advantage. We can learn from them, wrestle and grow with them. Struggling with difficulties makes us stronger, more capable, and more aware. This is not a time to settle; this is a time to reach for more. We can fix things that are broken and make the world better than it has ever been. This is our purpose. This is the task allotted us.

A parasite, psychic illness can never be more than an inferior substitute for a healthy life. Any power the virus has is stolen. Its powers are derivative. It is and will always be inferior to humans and the path with heart (Kornfield, 1993). Life and love are the superior way to walk through this world. More effective, more enjoyable, and longer lasting: love wins.

What are your pain and problems telling you? A better way beckons. Another world is possible. We can make our minds, hearts, and souls right by addressing these problems. We can do more than repair; we can rebuild and grow. This is the challenge before us now. Every fiber, every cell, every stitch of our being screams at us to fight this thing. Engage these problems as they were meant. No generation has ever had the opportunities laid before us now: to transform humankind and deliver the world to a higher order of being. The virus is testing us, probing our weaknesses and seeing what we are made of. Of late, we have done a lot of failing, and the short end of this path becomes more clear with each wayward misstep. Open your mind, open your heart, and try a few steps on the other path, toward sanity, reason, connection, caring, sustainability, survival, and yes, God. We are being called. Your higher nature yearns to unfold. Look within, and you will feel it. Follow this path, and you change the world.

We stand now at a crossroads between two fates that could not be more different. We can make this world into a living Hell, or we can live amazing lives, heal, grow, save a planet, and remake this world into a garden. We can descend into depravity and wickedness, or we can do what is needed and just and forge a new species: Homo Humanus. Human 2.0. The choice is ours. We were made for better things. We shall rise to this day, meet these challenges, defend the rights of all that live, and create a world better than given us. This is not some starry-eyed dream. This is the reality before us now. We have everything we need. We have the resources and the technology to make this world a sustainable paradise, a thriving planet with no poverty, hunger, or war. We lack only the will. The question is not, "What do we need to do?" The question is, "Will we do it?" This next century will be the demise of civilization and ruin of humankind, or it will be our finest hour. There are no other paths.

The universe is knocking ever louder at our door, demanding an answer: *Who are you? What is man?* We have many choices before us, but we have only one choice: Will we love one another? We will heal by caring for each other. We shall stand together, or we shall fall. It begins here. It begins now. We have a world of work to do. Our task is to dismantle this beast and remake this world.

Are you in?

References

117th Congress Second Session. (2022, Dec. 22). Final report, select committee to investigate the January 6th attack on the United States Capitol. *House Report 117*-663.
Abramson, L.Y., Metalsky, G.I., & Alloy, L.B. (1989). Hopelessness depression: A theory-based subtype of depression. *Psychological Review, 96*(2), 358-372.
Acemoglu, D. & Robinson, J.A. (2013). *Why nations fail: The origins of power, prosperity, and poverty.* New York: Currency.
Alighieri, D. (1320/2013). *The inferno.* CreateSpace.
Aristotle. (350 B.C.E./1926). *The Nicomachean ethics.* (H. Rackham, Trans.) London: W. Heinemann.
Attenborough, R. (Director, Producer), & Briley, J. (Writer). (1982). *Gandhi* [Film]. Columbia Pictures; EMI-Warner Distributors.
Axelrod, R., & Hamilton, W. D. (1981). The Evolution of Cooperation. *Science, 211*(4489), 1390-1396. https://doi.org/doi:10.1126/science.7466396
Bakan, J. (2004). *The corporation: The pathological pursuit of profit and power.* New York: Free Press.
Bandura, A. (1977). *Social learning theory.* Englewood Cliffs, NJ: Prentice-Hall.

Bosker, B. (2016, Nov.). The binge breaker. *The Atlantic.* https://www.theatlantic.com/magazine/archive/2016/11/the-binge-breaker/501122/

Cadwell, O.G. (2015). Literary fiction's influence on social cognitive brain activity. *Proceedings of The National Conference on Undergraduate Research (NCUR) 2015.* Eastern Washington University, April 16 -18, 2015

Calvin, W.H. (2002). *A brain for all seasons: Human evolution and abrupt climate change.* University of Chicago Press.

Carter-Scott, C. (1998). *If life is a game, these are the rules.* New York: Broadway.

Cipolletti, H., McFarlane, S., & Weissglass, C. (2016). The Moral Foreign-Language Effect. *Philosophical Psychology, 29*(1), 23-40. https://doi.org/10.1080/09515089.2014.993063

Darwin, C. (1871/1930). *The descent of man.* Watts & Co.

Dawkins, R. (1976). *The selfish gene.* New York: Oxford U. Press.

Desmettre T. (2020). Toxoplasmosis and behavioural changes. *Journal francais d'ophtalmologie, 43*(3), e89–e93. https://doi.org/10.1016/j.jfo.2020.01.001

Dominguez, J. & Robin, V. (1992). *Your money or your life: Transforming your relationship with money and achieving financial independence.* Penguin.

Douglas, K. M., Sutton, R. M., & Cichocka, A. (2017). The psychology of conspiracy theories. *Current Directions in Psychological Science 26*(6): 538-542. https://doi.org/10.1177/0963721417718261

Eisenhower, D. (1961, Jan. 17). *Farewell radio and television address to the American people.* Dwight D. Eisenhower Presidential Library. https://www.eisenhowerlibrary.gov/sites/default/files/file/farewell_address.pdf

Elkington, J. (1998). *Cannibals with forks: The triple bottom line of 21st-century business.* New Society Publishers.
Environmental Protection Agency (2022). *PFAS explained.* https://www.epa.gov/pfas/pfas-explained
Flegr, J., Zitková, Š., Kodym, P., & Frynta, D. (1996). Induction of changes in human behavior by the parasitic protozoan Toxoplasma gondii. *Parasitology, 113*(1), 49-54. https://doi.org/10.1017/S0031182000066269
Floyd, D., (2023, Jan. 23). Explaining the Trump tax reform plan. Investopedia. https://www.investopedia.com/taxes/trumps-tax-reform-plan-explained/
Fouts, R., Mills, S.T., & Routs, R. (1997). *Next of kin: My conversations with chimpanzees.* William Morrow.
Frank, T. (2004). *What's the matter with Kansas?: How conservatives won the heart of America* (1st ed.). Metropolitan Books.
Fromm, E. (1976). *To have or to be?* Harper & Row.
Gage, F.K. (2003). Brain repair yourself. *Scientific American, Special Issue, 289*(3), 46-53.
Gallup News. In depth: topics A to Z. *Guns.* (2023). https://news.gallup.com/poll/1645/guns.aspx
Graham, K. E. and C. Hobaiter (2023). Towards a great ape dictionary: Inexperienced humans understand common nonhuman ape gestures. *PLOS Biology* 21(1): e3001939.
Groeschel, C. (2021). *Winning the war in your mind.* Zondervan.
Harari, Yuval N. (2015). *Sapiens: A brief history of humankind.* Harper.
Hawken, P. (2010). *The ecology of commerce revised edition: A declaration of sustainability.* Harper Business.

Hawking, S.W. (1996). Academic lectures: *Life in the universe.* https://www.hawking.org.uk/in-words/lectures/life-in-the-universe

Hippocrates. (400 B.C.E./2015). On Airs, Waters, and Places (C.D. Adams, Trans.) *Complete Works of Hippocrates.* Delphi Classics.

Hobbes, T. (1651/2008). *Leviathan* (J. C. A. Gaskin, Ed.). Oxford.

Hollis, H. (2021). Readers' experiences of fiction and nonfiction influencing critical thinking. *Journal of Librarianship and Information Science, 0*(0), 09610006211053040. https://doi.org/10.1177/09610006211053040

Ion, R. & Kirsten, J. (2020, Nov.). Read it in books: Literary fiction as a tool to develop moral thinking in the educator. *Nurse Education Today Vol. 94,* Nov. 2020, 104538. https://doi.org/10.1016/j.nedt.2020.104538

Ismi, A. (2021, July 1). Ismi, A. 'Whoever controls the media, controls the mind.' *The Monitor.* https://monitormag.ca/articles/whoever-controls-the-media-controls-the-mind

Jackson, P. (2001). The Fellowship of the Ring. [Film]. New Line Cinema. Wing Nut Films.

Jackson, P. (2002). The Two Towers. [Film]. New Line Cinema. Wing Nut Films.

Jarvis, G. E. (2016). Early embryo mortality in natural human reproduction: What the data say. *F1000Res, 5,* 2765. https://doi.org/10.12688/f1000research.8937.2

Johnson SK, Fitza MA, Lerner DA, Calhoun DM, Beldon MA, Chan ET, Johnson PTJ. (2018). Risky business: Linking toxoplasma gondii infection and entrepreneurship behaviors across individuals and countries. *Proc. R. Soc. B 285:* 20180822. http://dx.doi.org/10.1098/rspb.2018.0822

Jung, C.G. (1995). The shadow. In Murray Stein (Ed.), *Jung on Evil* (1997, pp. 95-97). Princeton: Princeton Univ. Press.

Kidd, D. C., & Castano, E. (2013). Reading literary fiction improves theory of mind. *Science, 342(6156)*, 377-380. https://doi.org/doi:10.1126/science.1239918

Klaas, B. (2022). *Corruptible: Who gets power and how it changes us.* Scribner.

Kornfield, J. (1993). *A path with heart.* Bantam.

LaFleur, W. R. (1988). *Buddhism: A cultural perspective.* Prentice-Hall.

Lezak, M.D., Howieson, D.B., & Loring, D.W. (2004). *Neuropsychological assessment* (4th ed.) Oxford.

Libersat, F., Kaiser, M., & Emanuel, S. (2018). Mind control: How parasites manipulate cognitive functions in their insect hosts [Perspective]. *Frontiers in Psychology, 9.* https://doi.org/10.3389/fpsyg.2018.00572

Light, N., Fernbach, P. M., Rabb, N., Geana, M. V., & Sloman, S. A. (2022). Knowledge overconfidence is associated with anti-consensus views on controversial scientific issues. *Science Advances, 8*(29), eabo0038. https://doi.org/doi:10.1126/sciadv.abo0038

MacLean, P. D. (1990). *The triune brain in evolution: Role in paleocerebral functions.* Kluwer.

Maté, D. G. (2018). *In the realm of hungry ghosts.* Vermilion.

Mattis, J. (2022), *National Public Radio interview*, Sep. 2, 2019. https://www.npr.org/2019/09/02/756681750/jim-mattis-nations-with-allies-thrive-nations-without-allies-wither

Mobbs, D., Greicius, M.D., AbdelAzim, E., Menon, V. & Reiss, A. L. (2003). Humor modulates the mesolimbic reward centers. *Neuron, 40*, 1041-1048.

Mokili, J. L., Rohwer, F., & Dutilh, B. E. (2012). Metagenomics and future perspectives in virus discovery. *Current Opinion in Virology, 2*(1), 63-77.

National Institute of Standards and Technology (2023). *Backdoor.* Computer Security Resource Center: Glossary. https://csrc.nist.gov/glossary/term/backdoor#:~:text=Definition(s)%3A,is%20a%20potential%20security%20risk

Orwell, G. (1949/1987). *Nineteen eighty-four* (Complete ed.). London: Secker & Warburg.

Perry, B.D. (2001). The neurodevelopmental impact of violence in childhood. In D. Schetky and E.P. Benedek (Eds.), *Textbook of Child and Adolescent Forensic Psychiatry,* 221-238. Washington, D.C.: American Psychiatric Press. Washington, D.C.

Postman, N. (1985). *Amusing ourselves to death: Public discourse in the age of show business.* Viking Penguin.

Provine, R. (1996, Jan.-Feb.). Laughter: The study of laughter provides a novel approach to the mechanisms and evolution of vocal production, perception, and social behavior. *American Scientist, 84,* 38-45.

Rainville, P., Duncan, G.H., Price, D.D., Carrier, B., & Bushness, M.C. (1997). Pain affect encoded in human anterior cingulate but not somatosensory cortex. *Science, 277,* 968-971.

Reiner, R. (Director, Producer), & Sorkin, A. (Writer). (1995). *The American President* [Film]. Columbia Pictures; Universal Pictures; Castle Rock Entertainment; United International Pictures.

Roozenbeek, J. & S. van der Linden (2019). The fake news game: Actively inoculating against the risk of misinformation. *Journal of Risk Research* 22(5): 570-580.

Rowe, D.B. (2018). The \"novel\" approach: Using fiction to increase empathy. *Virginia Libraries, 63(1)*. DOI: http://doi.org/10.21061/valib.v63i1.1474

Russell, B. (1959). *Bertrand Russell - 'Love is wise, hatred is foolish'* [Video]. BBC interview on Face to Face.

Sagan, C. (1980). *Cosmos* (1st ed.). Random House.

Sakharov, A.D. (1958/1990). Radioactive carbon from nuclear explosions and non-threshold biological effects. *Science and Global Security, 1990, vol. I,* 175-187.

Seligman, M.E.P., Reivich, K., Jaycox, L., & Gillham, J. (1995). *The optimistic child.* Boston: Houghton Mifflin.

Serabian, R., & Foster, L. (2022). *Pro-PRC influence campaign expands to dozens of social media platforms, websites, and forums in at least seven languages*... https://www.mandiant.com/resources/blog/pro-prc-influence-campaign-expands-dozens-social-media-platforms-websites-and-forums

Stiglitz, J. (2019). Progressive capitalism is not an oxymoron: We can save our broken economic system from itself. *New York Times*, April 19, 2019.

Stirner, M. (1936/1962). Attributed in *Forbes Vol. 38.* Iss. 2 (1936) p. 18, and in *Lifetime Speaker's Encyclopedia* (1962) by Jacob Morton Braude, p. 275.

Sweitzer, G. (1988, Jun. 15). *Behaviorally transmitted psychic illness.* [Unpublished manuscript]. Library of Congress, Copyright Registration: TXU 328 939.

Sweitzer, G. (1989, May 26). *Behaviorally transmitted psychic illness.* [Unpublished manuscript]. Library of Congress, Copyright Registration: TXU 372 337.

Sweitzer, G. (2001). *Psychic illness: The rise and fall of evil on Earth* (1st ed.). Philadelphia: Xlibris.

Sweitzer, G. *Psychic illness: The rise and fall of evil on Earth* (2nd ed.). Manuscript in preparation.

Thoreau, H.D. (1854). *Walden.* Public domain.

Time Magazine (1938, May 9). *Anti-monopoly: Simple truths.* https://content.time.com/time/subscriber/article/0,33009,759590,00.html

Time Magazine (2022, June 9). *Exclusive: Iran steps up efforts to sow discord inside the U.S.* https://time.com/6071615/iran-disinformation-united-states/

Torrey, E. F., Bartko, J. J., & Yolken, R. H. (2012). Toxoplasma gondii and other risk factors for schizophrenia: An update. *Schizophrenia Bulletin, 38*(3), 642-647.

Trevelline, B. K., & Kohl, K. D. (2022). The gut microbiome influences host diet selection behavior. *Proceedings of the National Academy of Sciences, 119*(17), e2117537119. https://doi.org/doi:10.1073/pnas.2117537119

Truzzi, M. (1978). On the extraordinary: An attempt at clarification, *Zetetic Scholar, Vol. 1,* No. 1, p. 11.

van der Kolk, B.A. (1989). The compulsion to repeat the trauma: Re-enactment, revictimization, and masochism. *Psychiatric Clinics of North America, 12*(2), 389-411.

Veblen, T. (1899/1994). *The theory of the leisure class.* Penguin.

Watson, L. (1995). *Dark nature: A natural history of evil.* Harper Collins.

Wolfram, S. (2002). *A new kind of science.* Champaign, IL: Wolfram Media.

Zimmer, C. (2000). *Parasite rex: Inside the bizarre world of nature's most dangerous creatures.* Atria/Knopf.

About the Author

Gregory Sweitzer, MSW, MA, Psy.D., C.Psych., is a clinical and rehabilitation psychologist with over 40 years of psychotherapy experience. He began writing about psychic illness in 1988. His first book on this subject, *Psychic Illness: The Rise and Fall of Evil on Earth*, was published in 2001. The revised second edition of *Psychic Illness* is in preparation.

Manufactured by Amazon.ca
Bolton, ON

37821925R00136